Principles of Therapy in the Epilepsies

C.P. Panayiotopoulos

Principles of Therapy in the Epilepsies

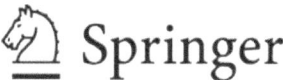 Springer

C.P. Panayiotopoulos MD, PhD, FRCP
Department of Clinical Neurophysiology and Epilepsies
St. Thomas Hospital
London SE1 7EH
United Kingdom
and
Department of Neurosciences
John Radcliffe Hospital
Oxford OX3 9DU
United Kingdom

ISBN 978-0-85729-008-3
Springer London Dordrecht Heidelberg New York

A catalogue record for this book is available from the British Library

Library of Congress Control Number: 2010936470

Cover design: eStudio Calamar S.L.

Printed on acid-free paper

Springer is part of Springer Science+Business Media (www.springer.com)

Contents

Preface

The aim of medicine is to diagnose, prevent, and treat (alleviate or cure) human diseases. Accurate diagnosis is a prerequisite and the golden rule for meaningful treatment. The systematic synthesis of evidence is the foundation of medical discoveries and of good clinical practice.

The traditional aim of therapy in epilepsies is total freedom from seizures with no clinically significant adverse effects. This has now been broadened to include optimal outcomes of health-related quality of life with regard to physical, mental, educational, social, and psychological functioning of the patient. This treatment goal cannot be achieved without a precise seizure and often syndrome diagnosis, which is a precondition for the success of therapeutic decisions. As in other areas of medicine, diagnostic precision in the epilepsies has become more refined over time and treatment has become more disease-specific.

The mainstay of treatment is usually with antiepileptic drugs (AEDs) in continuous prophylactic schemes. As with all drugs, AEDs may be therapeutic when appropriately used but they also possess toxic properties. A balance between the therapeutic and toxic effects of an AED is a primary responsibility and the crux of epilepsy management. Children, elderly people, women particularly of childbearing age, and patients with mental, physical, and other comorbidities are vulnerable and their treatment is more demanding.

An AED that is therapeutic in one type may be deleterious for another type of epileptic seizure. There are numerous examples in the literature of patients endangered by inappropriate use of AEDs either because of misdiagnosis or vague AED recommendations. Consider, for example, the aggravating effects of carbamazepine in patients with absences and myoclonic jerks, and a similar situation may occur with gabapentin, lamotrigine, and pregabalin given to patients with myoclonic jerks, as these agents may be pro-myoclonic.

Epilepsies are syndromes and diseases with multiple manifestations and causes that often demand disparate management strategies. This is exemplified by three common epileptic syndromes that comprise more than a third of all epilepsies: benign childhood focal seizures, juvenile myoclonic epilepsy (JME), and hippocampal epilepsy. They are entirely different in presentation, causes, investigative procedures, prognosis, and short- and long-term treatment strategies. Benign childhood focal seizures may or may not require medication for a few years, whereas appropriate AED treatment is lifelong in JME and neurosurgery may be the proper management of hippocampal epilepsy. Carbamazepine that often worsens JME is a beneficial drug in the other two conditions.

In clinical practice, a physician faces a colossal task not only to make the correct diagnosis but also to precisely identify which is the best therapeutic AED option. However, such judgement requires huge, extensive, continually updated and multilevel knowledge, which even expert clinical epileptologists may not have. Therefore, it is fundamental for physicians to be informed about the best existing evidence for AED treatment in clinical practice particularly with the multiplicity of therapies now available.

Recommendations and guidelines should be clear for each AED: what priority and for what type of seizures they are effective, potentially useful, ineffective, contraindicated, or harmful. Ideally, these recommendations should be based on unequivocal documentation but often this is limited to probable, possible, or purely anecdotal evidence. They are also influenced by commercial reputation rather than strict scientific evidence.

However, even in their best use, AEDs are ineffective for about 20% of patients. These patients are candidates for neurosurgical intervention and other pharmacological or nonpharmacological treatments.

Patients are entitled to the best possible information about their treatment, its purpose, efficacy, contraindications, adverse effects, and possibly its duration in order to make informed decisions. Inappropriate generalisation about the disease and its treatment is detrimental and does not meet the requirements of good clinical practice.

The aim of this concise booklet is to assist health care professionals in optimising the management of their patients with epileptic seizures by emphasising key points of clinical significance in an objective and updated evidence-based assessment.

C. P. Panayiotopoulos, MD, PhD, FRCP
June 2010
Oxford

Abbreviations

AAN-AES	American Academy of Neurology–American Epilepsy Society
ACTH	adrenocorticotrophic hormone
ADR	adverse drug reaction
AED	anti-epileptic drug
AHS	anticonvulsant hypersensitivity syndrome
CI	confidence interval
CNS	central nervous system
CONSERT	Consolidated Standards for Reporting of Trials
CRMP	collapsin response mediator protein
CYP	cytochrome P450
DSM	Diagnostic and Statistical Manual of Mental Dis-orders
EBM	evidence-based medicine
ECG	electrocardiogram
EEG	electroencephalogram
EMEA	European Medicines Agency
EURAP	European and International Registry of Anti-epileptic Drugs in Pregnancy
EUROCAT	European Surveillance of Congenital Ano-malies
FDA	US Food and Drug Administration
fMRI	functional magnetic resonance imaging
GABA	Gamma-aminobutyric acid
GTCS	generalised tonic–clonic seizure
HLA	human leukocyte antigen
ICH-E14	International Conference of Harmonisation topic E14
IGE	idiopathic generalised epilepsy
ILAE	International League Against Epilepsy
IQ	intelligence quotient
JME	juvenile myoclonic epilepsy
MCM	major congenital malformation
MEG	magnetoencephalography
MRI	magnetic resonance imaging
PI	package insert
RCT	randomised controlled trial
SmPC	Summary of Product Characteristics
SUDEP	sudden unexpected death in epilepsy
SV2A	synaptic vesicle protein 2A
TDM	therapeutic drug monitoring
UGT	uridine diphosphate glucuronosyltransferase
VGSC	voltage gated sodium channel
VNS	vagus nerve stimulation

Introduction

The traditional aim of therapy in epilepsies is total freedom from seizures with no clinically significant adverse effects. This has now been broadened to include optimal outcomes of health-related quality of life with regard to physical, mental, educational, social and psychological functioning of the patient. The mainstay of treatment is usually with anti-epileptic drugs (AEDs) in continuous prophylactic schemes. However, AEDs are ineffective for about 20% of patients. These patients are candidates for neurosurgical interventions, other pharmacological or non-pharmacological treatments.

A prerequisite for any treatment is that the patient truly suffers epileptic seizures; a quarter of patients treated for 'epilepsy' do not suffer genuine epileptic seizures.[1,2]

Correct seizure and often syndrome diagnosis is a precondition for the success of therapeutic decisions because the choice of AED primarily depends on seizure type, whereas length of treatment is mainly determined by syndrome type.

Anti-epileptic Drug Prophylactic Treatment

AED treatment is the mainstay of the management of epilepsies. The laudable aim is freedom from seizures with minimal, if any, adverse drug reactions (ADRs). This is achieved in about 50–70% of patients with a single, appropriately selected AED at target therapeutic doses. This seizure-free rate varies significantly with seizure type and epileptic syndrome. Polytherapy should be avoided if possible, but it is inevitable in about 30–50% of patients who fail to respond to single-drug therapy. Freedom of seizures should not be pursued at any cost and, in particular, at the expense of ADRs.

There is no point in treating epilepsy at the expense of drug-induced disease.

For some patients, a few minor and often harmless seizures may be allowed to occur instead of increasing the number of AEDs or their doses, which may jeopardise the quality of life of the patient. The identification of ADRs, although sometimes difficult, is a crucial part of the management.

Useful information

The 'package insert' (FDA in the USA) and the 'summary of product characteristics' (EMEA in the EU) are the most complete single sources of information on a drug. The package insert can be obtained from http://dailymed.nlm.nih.gov/dailymed/about.cfm. The summary of package characteristics can be obtained in any European language from http://www.emea.europa.eu/htms/human/epar/a.htm. In UK these are also available from http://emc.medicines.org.uk

The drug treatment of epilepsies requires thorough knowledge of the AEDs with regard to seizure-specific efficacy, acute and chronic ADRs, pharmacokinetics, doses and titration, drug interactions and contraindications. This information is widely available in books, journal reviews, manufacturers' prescribing information and credible internet sources.

As with all drugs, AEDs may be therapeutic when appropriately used (Table 1.1), but they also possess toxic properties (Table 1.2). A balance between the therapeutic and toxic effects of an AED is a primary responsibility and the crux of epilepsy management. This treatment goal cannot be achieved satisfactorily without a thorough evaluation of the patient's seizures, medical history, possible co-medication for other diseases and the individual patient's circumstances.

Efficacy of main AEDs in seizure types

AED	Focal seizures (simple or complex)	Secondarily GTCSs	Primarily GTCSs	Myoclonic jerks	Absence seizures
Carbamazepine	Effective	Effective	Effective	–[†]	–[†]
Clobazam[‡]	Effective	Effective	Effective?	Effective?	Effective?
Clonazepam[¶]	Effective?	Effective?	Ineffective?	Effective	Effective
Eslicarbazepine	Effective	Effective	Unknown	Unknown	Unknown
Ethosuximide	–	–	–	Effective?[§]	Effective
Gabapentin	Effective	Effective	–	–[¶¶]	May exaggerate
Lacosamide	Effective	Effective	Unknown	Unknown	Unknown
Lamotrigine	Effective	Effective	Effective	May exaggerate**	Effective
Levetiracetam	Effective	Effective	Effective	Effective	Effective[††]
Oxcarbazepine	Effective	Effective	Effective	–[‡‡]	–[‡‡]
Phenobarbital	Effective	Effective	Effective	Effective	–
Phenytoin	Effective	Effective	Effective	–	–
Pregabalin	Effective	Effective	–	Exaggerates[¶¶]	–
Tiagabine	Effective	Effective	–	–	Exaggerates
Topiramate	Effective	Effective	Effective	Effective?	Effective?
Valproate	Effective	Effective	Effective	Effective	Effective
Vigabatrin	Effective	Effective	–	–	Exaggerates
Zonisamide	Effective	Effective	Effective?[§§]	Effective?[§§]	Effective?[§§]

Table 1.1 This table is based predominantly on information obtained from the SmPCs[3–19] and PIs. AEDs in italics are, in general, contraindicated for the treatment of idiopathic generalised epilepsies. However, carbamazepine, oxcarbazepine and phenytoin may be used in the rare pure forms of primarily generalised tonic–clonic seizures (GTCSs). –, the cited AED is not indicated for this seizure type, either because it is not licensed or it is ineffective or may exaggerate the seizure. [†]According to the SmPC 'carbamazepine is not usually effective in absences and myoclonic seizures. Moreover, anecdotal evidence suggests that seizure exacerbation may occur in patients with atypical absences'. However, many observational reports have shown the deteriorating effect of carbamazepine in these types of seizure.[20–25] [‡]Clobazam is licensed only as adjunctive therapy in 'epilepsy'. Its efficacy is not the same as that of clonazepam. It may be more efficacious in focal than generalised epilepsies.[26–28] [¶]Clonazepam is licensed for any type of epileptic seizure, but it is mainly used as one of the most efficacious AEDs in myoclonic jerks. It may not suppress GTCSs of juvenile myoclonic epilepsy and patients may be deprived of the warning jerks, which herald the onset of GTCS.[29] [§]Ethosuximide may be effective in negative myoclonus.[30] **Lamotrigine may aggravate myoclonic jerks in juvenile myoclonic epilepsy and some progressive myoclonic epilepsies.[25,31–34] [††]The effect of levetiracetam on absences is not well documented, although clinical series have shown a significant beneficial effect in childhood and juvenile absence epilepsy.[35,36] [‡‡]Oxcarbazepine, like carbamazepine, may aggravate myoclonic jerks[37] and absence seizures.[38,39] [¶¶]Myoclonus is a treatment-emergent type of seizure in patients with focal seizures treated with pregabalin as an adjunctive medication[40] or even in non-epileptic patients receiving this drug for pain relief.[41] Gabapentin may have a similar promyoclonic effect.[24,42] This may signify the need for extreme caution in the use of pregabalin and gabapentin in epilepsies with myoclonus. [§§]Zonisamide, although licensed for focal seizures only, appears to be a broad-spectrum AED.[43]

Main adverse reactions of AEDs, which may sometimes be serious and rarely life threatening

AED	Main adverse reactions	Life threatening
Carbamazepine	Idiosyncratic (rash), sedation, headache, ataxia, nystagmus, diplopia, tremor, impotence, hyponatraemia, cardiac arrhythmia*	AHS[†], hepatic failure, haematological
Clobazam	Severe sedation, fatigue, drowsiness, behavioural and cognitive impairment, restlessness, aggressiveness, hypersalivation and coordination disturbances. Tolerance and withdrawal syndrome	No
Clonazepam	As for clobazam	No
Eslicarbazepine	Idiosyncratic (rash), dizziness, somnolence, headache, ataxia, inattention, diplopia, tremor, nausea, vomiting, hyponatraemia, PR prolongation in ECG	No
Ethosuximide	Idiosyncratic (rash), gastrointestinal disturbances, anorexia, weight loss, drowsiness, photophobia, headache	AHS[†], renal and hepatic failure, haematological
Gabapentin	Weight gain, peripheral oedema, behavioural changes, impotence, viral infection*	Acute pancreatitis, hepatitis, Stevens–Johnson syndrome, acute renal failure[‡]
Lacosamide	Dizziness, headache, diplopia, nausea, vomiting, blurred vision, PR prolongation in ECG	No
Lamotrigine	Idiosyncratic (rash), tics, insomnia, dizziness, diplopia, headache, ataxia, asthenia*	AHS[†], hepatic failure, haematological
Levetiracetam	Irritability, behavioural and psychotic changes, asthenia, dizziness, somnolence, headache*	Hepatic failure, hepatitis[‡]
Oxcarbazepine	Idiosyncratic (rash), headache, dizziness, weakness, nausea, somnolence, ataxia and diplopia, hyponatraemia*	AHS[†], haematological
Phenobarbital	Idiosyncratic (rash), severe drowsiness, sedation, impairment of cognition and concentration, hyperkinesia and agitation in children, shoulder–hand syndrome	AHS[†], hepatic failure, haematological
Phenytoin	Idiosyncratic (rash), ataxia, drowsiness, lethargy, sedation, encephalopathy, gingival hyperplasia, hirsutism, dysmorphism, rickets, osteomalacia	AHS[†], hepatic failure, haematological
Pregabalin	Weight gain, myoclonus, dizziness, somnolence, ataxia, confusion*	Renal failure, congestive heart failure, AHS[†,‡]

Table 1.2 *Continued on next page.*

Main adverse reactions of AEDs, which may sometimes be serious and rarely life threatening

AED	Main adverse reactions	Life threatening
Tiagabine	Stupor or spike–wave stupor, weakness*	Status epilepticus
Topiramate	Somnolence, anorexia, fatigue, nervousness, difficulty with concentration/attention, memory impairment, psychomotor slowing, metabolic acidosis, weight loss, language dysfunction, renal calculi, acute angle-closure glaucoma and other ocular abnormalities, paraesthesiae*	Hepatic failure, anhidrosis
Valproate	Nausea, vomiting, dyspepsia, weight gain, tremor, hair loss, hormonal in women*	Hepatic and pancreatic failure
Vigabatrin	Irreversible visual field defects, fatigue, weight gain	No
Zonisamide	Idiosyncratic, drowsiness, anorexia, irritability, photosensitivity, weight loss, renal calculi*	AHS[†], anhidrosis

Table 1.2 This table is based predominantly on information obtained from the SmPCs[3–19] and PIs. It is an assessment of common ADRs and/or those of clinical importance. It is not an exhaustive list of all ADRs; for these, readers should refer to the relevant chapters of *Epileptic Syndromes and Their Treatment*[282] and, mainly, to the SmPC or PI of each AED. For more details, see "Considerations of adverse antiepileptic drug reactions in the treatment of epilepsies" and the pharmacopoeia. *FDA warning for suicidal ideation (see below, "Life-Threatening ADRs"). [†]AHS, anticonvulsant hypersensitivity syndrome. [‡]Post-marketing experience.

Patients and parents should be well informed about the purpose of AED medication, and its efficacy, ADRs and possible length of treatment. Otherwise, there are failures in compliance, disenchantment and breaking down of patient/physician trust.

Special groups of patients with epileptic disorders require particular attention and management. Children, elderly people, women (particularly of childbearing age) and patients with mental, physical and other comorbidities are vulnerable and their treatment is more demanding. A special section on women (see chapter 2) and the elderly (see chapter 3) has been added in this revision.

Key points of AED treatment

- The aim of AED treatment is to achieve seizure-freedom without ADRs.
- The first-option AED is the most likely to be efficacious and the most unlikely to cause ADRs.
- The correct AED dose is the smallest one that achieves seizure control without ADRs.
- An AED appropriate for one type of seizure may be deleterious for another type.
- Titrating to the limit of tolerability may improve AED efficacy, but often at the cost of ADRs.
- Optimal efficacy of an AED may be lost by exceeding tolerability limits.

Cost should not be an issue in medicine, but with most of the global population living in poverty and often in conditions of starvation, options are frequently limited to the older AEDs, which are often life-saving agents.

Clarifications on terminology of AED treatment

Efficacy is not synonymous with effectiveness.

Efficacy is the ability of a medication to produce a clinically measurable beneficial effect aiming at seizure freedom.[44] It is a relative term defined by the designers of a study, but is usually a specific effect of a treatment. A drug can be highly efficacious yet not very clinically useful; i.e., not clinically effective.

There is no formal definition or the exact limits of the term *'spectrum of efficacy'*. In clinical practice, broad spectrum AEDs are those that are efficacious in all or most of focal and generalised epileptic seizures, while narrow spectrum refers to those with efficacy in one or few types of either focal or generalised seizures.

Effectiveness, in contrast to efficacy, is meant to be a more pragmatic measure that addresses the utility of a drug as it is actually employed in practice.[44,45] Effectiveness encompasses both AED efficacy and tolerability, as reflected in retention on treatment.[44] Effectiveness encompasses many potential components including tolerability, cognition, mood or quality of life.

Tolerability involves the incidence, severity and impact of ADRs.[44]

Thus, an AED efficacious in controlling seizures may not be effective because of high incidence or severe ADRs as, for example, with vigabatrin in focal seizures because of irreversible visual field defects or felbamate, which has not been licensed by the EMEA because of a high incidence of aplastic anaemia and hepatic failure.

ADRs are not synonymous with adverse drug effects or side effects.

According to the International Conference on Harmonisation of Definitions and Standards:

> *ADR is a response to a drug which is noxious and unintended, and which occurs at doses normally used for prophylaxis, diagnosis, or therapy of disease, or for modification of physiological function. The phrase 'responses to a medicinal product' means that a causal relationship between a medicinal product and an adverse event is at least a possibility.*
>
> *An adverse event is any untoward medical occurrence in a patient administered a medicinal product and which does not necessarily have to have a causal relationship with this treatment. An adverse event can therefore be any unfavorable and unintended sign (for example, an abnormal laboratory finding), symptom, or disease temporally associated with the use of a medicinal product, whether or not considered related to this medicinal product.*

See www.fda.gov/cber/gdlns/ichexrep.htm.

Choosing the best AED option

The ideal profile of a first-choice AED in the prophylactic treatment of epilepsies is determined by a number of factors (Table 1.3).

The importance of these factors varies significantly according to whether the AED is used in monotherapy or polytherapy.

Seizure specificity

The first-choice AED should primarily be in accord with the seizure type. Some AEDs may be very efficacious in some epileptic seizures and syndromes, but contraindicated in others (Table 1.1). Carbamazepine, for example, is a first-choice AED in focal seizures but should be avoided in idiopathic generalised epilepsies (IGEs).

Strength of efficacy

The more efficacious a drug the more likely it is to control seizures. Seizure-free status is the ultimate, often achievable, goal of treatment. That an AED may achieve more than 50% seizure reduction is not the best option, although this is a common outcome measurement in randomised controlled trials (RCTs).

Spectrum of efficacy

This is significant in the treatment of patients when the differentiation between focal and generalised epileptic seizures cannot be certain. In such cases broad-spectrum AEDs are recommended (Table 1.1), which are those that are efficacious in a wide range of focal and generalised epileptic seizures, and include valproate, levetiracetam, lamotrigine, topiramate and zonisamide.

Useful clinical notes

Women are more sensitive than men to specific ADRs
- Valproate: reproductive ADRs.
- AEDs that are associated with weight gain (Table 1.4): polycystic ovarian syndrome.
- AEDs that are associated with aesthetic changes (phenytoin).
- AEDs that are associated with increased risk of teratogenicity (pregnancy category D).
- AEDs that interact with hormonal contraception or pregnancy (enzyme inducers and lamotrigine).

Children are more susceptible than adults to specific ADRs
- Valproate: hepatotoxicity.
- Lamotrigine: AHS.
- Phenobarbital: hyperkinetic behaviour and cognitive impairment.
- Topiramate and zonisamide: hypohidrosis (anhidrosis).

Safety, tolerability and adverse reactions

These vary significantly between AEDs (Table 1.2) Adverse drug reactions may outweigh any beneficial effect achieved by reduction of the seizures. Currently, with so many efficacious AEDs, it is possible to avoid those with significant ADRs and particularly those associated with sometimes fatal ADRs, teratogenicity or significant impairment of quality of life. Carbamazepine, lamotrigine, oxcarbazepine, phenytoin, phenobarbital and zonisamide are associated with frequent idiosyncratic reactions and anticonvulsant hypersensitivity syndrome (AHS), which may be fatal. Women, children and elderly patients are more vulnerable to ADRs from certain AEDs; for example, valproate in babies and women of childbearing age. In children, documented or potential ADRs on growth, height and weight should be meticulously considered. Treatment-emergent weight changes should also be a significant concern (Table 1.4).

Clinical pharmacokinetics[47–49]

Pharmacokinetics is the study of the time course of a drug and its metabolites in humans. Absorption, distribution, metabolism and excretion are the primary parameters of pharmacokinetics and these significantly influence efficacy, ADRs and interactions with hormones and other drugs. AEDs with high pharmacokinetic profile scores should be preferred (Table 1.5).[47–49] Most commonly used AEDs are eliminated through hepatic metabolism catalysed by cytochrome P450 (CYP)

Properties of AEDs to consider in prioritising their use	
• Seizure specificity	• Pharmacokinetics
• Strength of efficacy	• Phamacodynamics
• Spectrum of efficacy	• Drug–drug interactions
• Safety	• Mechanisms of action
• Tolerability	• Speed of titration (time needed to reach effective dose)
• Adverse reactions (particularly if these are severe and life threatening)	• Frequency of administration and ease of use
• Need for laboratory testing	• Cost of treatment

Table 1.3 Factors highlighted in red are of particular importance in polytherapy.

Main AEDs that are likely to affect body weight	
The risks of obesity are emphasised routinely in the media in the USA, UK and other industrialised countries where obesity has become epidemic	
Patients, particularly women (e.g. see increased risk for polycystic ovarian syndrome), should be informed of the following AEDs that are likely to cause weight gain:	
• Gabapentin	• Valproate
• Pregabalin	• Vigabatrin
Significant weight loss, which can be relentless, may be caused by:	
• Topiramate	• Zonisamide
Note: Levetiracetam may be associated with a decrease[46] or increase of body weight	

Table 1.4 This table is based predominantly on information obtained from the SmPCs[7,10,14,16–19] and PIs.

and uridine diphosphate glucuronosyltransferase (UGT) enzymes (Table 1.6). Hepatic enzyme modifiers have low priority over others, particularly in patients who are receiving co-medications. Carbonic anhydrase inhibitors (Table 1.7), such as topiramate, reduce urinary citrate excretion and increase urinary pH, resulting in an increased risk of metabolic acidosis (which increases the risk for nephrolithiasis and osteomalacia/osteoporosis, and reduces growth rates in children). Different formulations of the same AED may have different bioavailability, which explains the loss of efficacy or emerging signs of toxicity when switching from one preparation to another. This is also the case with some controlled-release formulations such as that of carbamazepine, which has a more variable bioavailability than the conventional forms. Major metabolic pathways and elimination of AEDs are important to consider, particularly in patients with any type of hepatic or renal impairment (Table 1.8).

Hepatic enzyme induction and inhibition

Hepatic enzyme induction stimulate the production and increase the amount of CYP enzymes (Table 1.6). This, in turn, increases the rate of metabolism of drugs metabolised by the CYP enzymes, thus resulting in lower plasma concentrations. Conversely, hepatic enzyme inducers may increase the bioavailability of drugs that require metabolism for their activation. The effect of hepatic induction, unlike hepatic inhibition, persists for several days following the withdrawal of the enzyme inducer drug.

Useful clinical notes

For AEDs that are eliminated renally (Table 1.8), either completely unchanged (e.g. gabapentin, pregabalin and vigabatrin) or mainly unchanged (e.g. lacosamide, levetiracetam and topiramate), the pharmacokinetic variability is small and usually predictable. However, the dose-dependent absorption of gabapentin increases its pharmacokinetic variability. Interactions with other drugs can affect their plasma concentration markedly, and individual factors such as age, pregnancy and renal function will contribute to the pharmacokinetic variability of all renally eliminated AEDs.

Pharmacokinetic profile rating of AEDs

Superior

Lacosamide (96), levetiracetam (96), vigabatrin (96), gabapentin (89), pregabalin (89)

Moderate

Topiramate (79), ethosuximide (77), oxcarbazepine (77), lamotrigine (73)

Inferior

Tiagabine (67), zonisamide (67), phenobarbital (57), valproate (52), carbamazepine (50), phenytoin (50)

Table 1.5 Numbers in parenthesis are the scores derived from a semi-quantitative rating system based on 16 pharmacokinetic parameters. The maximum possible score is 100.[48,49]

If the affected drug has an active metabolite the impact of an inducer may be reduced, but this depends on the subsequent metabolism of the metabolites; for example, induction may increase metabolite concentrations and enhance toxicity without elevation of the parent drug.

Enzyme inducers, by speeding up the elimination of other substances that are metabolised in the liver, have significant disadvantages:

- Drug–drug interactions make them undesirable in polytherapy.
- Some hormones critical to sexual function are metabolised in the liver and levels of these hormonal substances may be reduced. Thus, long use of hepatic enzyme inducers can lead to significant changes in sex hormones in women and may potentially result in long-term endocrine effects in children. Furthermore, CYP3A4 enzyme inducers increase clearance of oestrogen and also of the progestational component of hormonal contraception, thus decreasing their plasma levels and effectiveness.
- Increased metabolism of vitamin D, which is metabolised through the liver, may result in hypocalcaemia, osteomalacia (rickets in children) and osteoporosis. It is reasonable to advise taking calcium and vitamin D supplements.

AEDs that are hepatic enzyme inducers and/or inhibitors

AED	Enzyme induced	Enzyme inhibited
Carbamazepine	CYP2C, CYP3A, CYP1A2, microsomal epoxide hydrolases, UGTs	–
Lamotrigine	UGTs	–
Oxcarbazepine	CYP3A4, UGTs	CYP2C19
Phenobarbital	CYP2C, CYP3A, microsomal epoxide hydrolases, UGTs	–
Phenytoin	CYP2C, CYP3A, microsomal epoxide hydrolases, UGTs	–
Topiramate	Dose-dependent enzyme inducer CYP3A4, β-oxidation	CYP2C19
Valproate	–	CYP2C9, microsomal epoxide hydrolases, UGTs

CYP (cytochrome P450 system) is a superfamily of isoenzymes that are responsible for the oxidative metabolism of many drugs, exogenous compounds and endogenous substrates. They are located in the membranes of the smooth endoplasmic reticulum, mainly of the liver. CYP enzymes are classified into families (designated by the first Arabic number), subfamilies (designated by the capital letter after the Arabic number) and isoenzymes according to the similarities in their amino acid sequences

UGTs (uridine diphosphate glucuronosyltransferases) are a superfamily of enzymes that are responsible for the formation of hydrophilic drug metabolites, which are mainly excreted via renal or biliary routes. They catalyse the glucuronidation of drugs and endogenous substrates. They are located in the endoplasmic reticulum of cells in the liver, kidneys and other organs, including the brain. Glucuronidation, mainly hepatic glucuronidation, represents one of the main detoxification pathways in humans

Table 1.6

Hepatic enzyme inhibition usually occurs because of competition at the enzyme site.

In enzyme inhibition, the added drug inhibits or blocks drug-metabolising enzymes, which in turn decreases the rate of metabolism of the other drug, causing higher plasma concentrations.

Carbonic anhydrase inhibitors

Carbonic anhydrase inhibitors (Table 1.7) reduce urinary citrate excretion and increase urinary pH. They need particular attention in clinical practice because they may induce hyperchloraemic, non-anion gap, metabolic acidosis (i.e. decreased plasma bicarbonate below the normal reference range in the absence of respiratory alkalosis). Chronic, untreated metabolic acidosis may:

- increase the risk of nephrolithiasis or nephrocalcinosis
- result in osteomalacia (rickets in children) and/or osteoporosis with an increased risk for fractures
- reduce growth rates in children and eventually decrease the maximal height achieved.

The effect of topiramate and zonisamide on growth and bone-related sequelae is unknown and has not been systematically investigated.

Carbonic anhydrase inhibitors

Acetazolamide
Sulthiame
Topiramate
Zonisamide

Table 1.7

Major metabolic and elimination pathways of AEDs

Hepatic	
Carbamazepine	Phenobarbital
Clobazam	Phenytoin
Clonazepam	Tiagabine
Ethosuximide	Topiramate
Lamotrigine	Valproate
Oxcarbazepine	Zonisamide
Renal	
Gabapentin	Pregabalin
Lacosamide	Vigabatrin
Levetiracetam	

Table 1.8

Useful clinical notes

AEDs that are carbonic anhydrase inhibitors

Avoid concomitant administration of carbonic anhydrase inhibitors because of the increased risk of:

- metabolic acidosis
- heat-related adverse events during exercise and exposure to warm environments
- nephrolithiasis.

Do not use them with anticholinergic drugs or a ketogenic diet.

Diseases or therapies that predispose to acidosis, such as renal disease, severe respiratory disorders, status epilepticus, diarrhoea, surgery, ketogenic diet or certain drugs, may add to the bicarbonate-lowering effects of carbonic anhydrase inhibitors.

Manifestations of acute or chronic metabolic acidosis may include hyperventilation, non-specific symptoms such as fatigue and anorexia, or more severe sequelae, including cardiac arrhythmias or stupor.

Pharmacodynamics

Pharmacodynamics refers to the biochemical and physiological effects of drugs and their mechanisms of action. They may be additive, synergistic or antagonistic. They may be beneficial, detrimental or both, as exemplified by lamotrigine combined with valproate (increased therapeutic efficacy but also increased risk of ADRs and teratogenicity).

Drug–drug interactions

These refer to phamacokinetic and pharmacodynamic changes that occur through concomitant use of drugs (Table 1.6). They are frequent causes of therapeutic failures and ADRs. Most AEDs are associated with a wide range of drug interactions, including hepatic enzyme induction and inhibition, and protein-binding displacement. Anticipation of induction or inhibition interactions and careful clinical monitoring may alleviate potential problems. Occasionally, drug–drug interactions may be beneficial (increased effectiveness, reduced risk of unwanted adverse reactions or both).

Useful clinical notes

Pharmacokinetic and pharmacodynamic interactions as exemplified by lamotrigine

Lamotrigine demands significant clinical attention in polytherapy, hormonal contraception and pregnancy.

Lamotrigine is metabolised predominantly in the liver by glucuronic acid conjugation. The major metabolite is an inactive 2-*N*-glucuronide conjugate. UGT1A4 is the major enzyme responsible for *N*-glucuronidation of lamo-trigine. Lamotrigine is a weak UGT enzyme inducer.

Lamotrigine dose and titration schemes are different in co-medication with valproate or enzyme inducers. The reason for this is that valproate is a potent inhibitor of UGT-dependent metabolism of lamotrigine, whereas enzyme-inducer AEDs are potent inducers of UGT-dependent metabolism of lamotrigine.

Lamotrigine undergoes important changes in conjunction with initiation or withdrawal of hormonal contraception and before, during and after pregnancy. The reason for this is that pregnancy and hormonal contraception significantly lower (by more than half) lamotrigine levels. Patients may suffer breakthrough seizures mainly during the first trimester of pregnancy (if lamotrigine levels are not corrected) or have toxic effects post partum (if lamotrigine levels had been adjusted during pregnancy but not after delivery).[50]

Lamotrigine also has significant pharmacodynamic interactions with valproate that are beneficial (increased therapeutic efficacy),[51] although they may also be detrimental as result of an increased risk of ADRs[52] and teratogenicity.[53]

Mechanisms of action

Mechanisms of action vary significantly among AEDs (Table 1.9)[54–57] and they have not been fully elucidated for most of them. The main mechanisms of action of the available AEDs are thought to be:

- blockade of voltage-dependent ion channels (K^+, Na^+ and Ca^{2+} channels)
- increasing the activity of the inhibitory GABA-ergic system

• decreasing the activity of the excitatory glutamatergic system.

The mechanism of action of levetiracetam – modulating the function of the synaptic vesicle 2A protein (SV2A) – is likely to be distinct from that of all other AEDs[58]. Lacosamide also has novel mechanisms of action (see Figure 1.1).

In clinical practice, knowledge about the mechanism of action is significant particularly in the treatment of seiz-ure types with known pathophysiology; for example, pri-marily GABA-ergic AEDs such as tiagabine and vigabatrin are contra-indicated in absence seizures that are facilitated by $GABA_B$ activation. Furthermore, in polytherapy, combining AEDs with the same action is ill-advised because their combination is unlikely to have a better success and more likely to have additive ADRs.[59,60]

Need for as little titration as possible

AEDs of fast titration should have priority over those demanding slower titration (Table 1.10). Slow titration may mean more seizures (which may also be hazardous)

AEDs: main mechanisms of actions
Blocking voltage-dependent Na⁺ channels ($\downarrow$Na⁺)
• Carbamazepine
• Lamotrigine
• Oxcarbazepine
• Phenytoin
Multiple, mainly or including blocking voltage-dependent Na⁺ channels
• Phenobarbital ($\downarrow$Na⁺, $\downarrow$Ca²⁺, $\uparrow$GABA, $\downarrow$glutamate)
• Topiramate ($\downarrow$Na⁺, $\downarrow$Ca²⁺, $\uparrow$GABA, $\downarrow$glutamate)
• Valproate ($\downarrow$Na⁺, $\downarrow$Ca²⁺, $\uparrow$GABA, $\downarrow$glutamate)
• Zonisamide ($\downarrow$Na⁺, $\downarrow$Ca²⁺)
Increasing GABA inhibition ($\uparrow$GABA)
• Clobazam (GABA$_A$)
• Clonazepam (GABA$_A$)
• Tiagabine (inhibitor of GABA uptake into neurones and glial cells)
• Vigabatrin (selective, irreversible GABA transaminase inhibitor)
Blocking T-type Ca²⁺ channels ($\downarrow$Ca²⁺)
• Ethosuximide
Modifying Ca²⁺ channels and neurotransmitter release
• Gabapentin
• Pregabalin
Novel: binding to synaptic vesicle protein SV2A
• Levetiracetam
Novel: (1) selectively enhancing slow inactivation voltage-gated Na⁺ channels; (2) may be binding to collapsin response mediator protein-2 (CRMP-2)*
• Lacosamide

Table 1.9 Based on data taken from the SmPCs[3–19] and PIs and references.[54–57] *More recent experiments did not confirm binding of lacosamide with CRMP-2.

and be more difficult for patients to follow (compliance may be lessened). Starting with small doses and a slow titration rate is mandated for lamotrigine (increased risk of skin rash) and topiramate (increased risk of cognitive impairment), which need 6–8 weeks in order to reach reasonable therapeutic levels. It is of less concern in others, such as gabapentin and levetiracetam (Table 1.10)

Need for less laboratory testing and other monitoring (Table 1.11)

Patients on AEDs may need laboratory testing and other monitoring for: (1) the detection of ADRs associated with certain AEDs, such as oxcarbazepine or valproate; and (2) therapeutic drug monitoring (TDM), as for lamotrigine in pregnancy and hormonal contraception, and carbamazepine, oxcarbazepine, lamotrigine, topiramate and zonisamide in co-medication when polytherapy is needed or for co-morbid disorders. More laboratory testing may also mean less compliance, more expense and more uncomfortable situations for patients.

Frequency of administration and ease of use

AEDs that need dosing more than twice a day are not practical for patient use and may lessen compliance. The frequency of administration is often determined by the plasma half-life. Most AEDs are given twice daily. Phenytoin and phenobarbital are the more advantageous, needing one dose per day before sleep. Doses three-times per day may be needed for gabapentin and sometimes for carbamazepine, pregabalin and oxcarbazepine. In large doses, some AEDs may need to be given three times daily to avoid ADRs associated with high peak plasma concentrations.

Mechanism of action of lacosamide

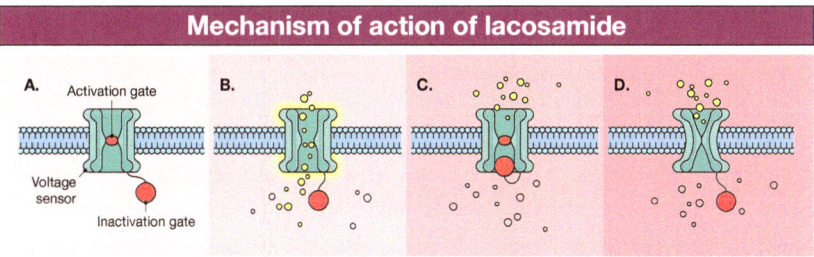

Figure 1.1 (A) Voltage gated sodium channel (B) activated VGSC (C) traditional fast inactivation as with most AEDs and (D) slow inactivation as with lacosamide.

Titration of AEDs: the recommendation of 'start low and go slow' is AED dependent

AEDs that do not need slow titration; the first dose may be therapeutic[7,10]	AEDs that need very slow titration of 6–8 weeks to reach therapeutic dose[9,12,16]
Gabapentin*	Lamotrigine
Levetiracetam*,†	Phenobarbital
	Topiramate

Table 1.10 All other AEDs need slow titration of approximately 4 weeks. *Results from studies on adjunctive therapy.[7,10] †Slow titration may be needed when used as adjunctive therapy.[10]

Patient-friendly formulations are particularly important for children or adults who may have difficulties in swallowing tablets or capsules, some of which may be very large.

Parenteral formulations are significant when oral administration is temporarily not feasible.[282] Levetiracetam and lacosamide are the only newer AEDs with oral and parenteral formulations.

Useful clinical note

Dosing of AEDs in children
Young children metabolise AEDs more rapidly than adults and therefore require more frequent dosing and a higher amount per kilogram of body weight.

Cost of treatment

Cost is often a significant factor, particularly in resource-poor countries and when medication is not freely provided by national health systems or personal health insurance. All newer AEDs are very expensive in relation to older generation AEDs.

Newest generation AEDs licensed in the treatment of focal epilepsies: lacosamide and eslicarbazepine

Despite the explosion of new therapeutic options in the last 15 years, there is still a great need for new AEDs for improving seizure control and the quality of life of patients with treatment-resistant epilepsies.

Lacosamide (Vimpat®) is the first of the newest AEDs to be licensed for prescribing this year by the EMEA and FDA. Lacosamide is indicated for the adjunctive treatment of focal seizures with or without secondarily generalised tonic–clonic seizures in patients with epilepsy aged 16 years (17 years in the

Need for laboratory testing and TDM

Minimal	Maximal
Clobazam	Carbamazepine (haematological toxicity, hyponatraemia, TDM)
Clonazepam	Lamotrigine (idiosyncratic reactions, TDM)
Gabapentin	Oxcarbazepine (hyponatraemia)
Lacosamide	Phenytoin (haematological and liver toxicity, TDM)
Levetiracetam	Topiramate (metabolic acidosis, TDM)
Pregabalin	Valproate (hepatotoxicity)
Tiagabine	Zonisamide (metabolic acidosis, TDM)

Table 1.11 TDM, therapeutic drug monitoring.

USA) and older.[8] The indication has been granted for the oral tablet, oral syrup and intravenous formulations.[8]

This decision is supported by data from three multicentre, double-blind, placebo-controlled clinical trials that evaluated the efficacy, safety and tolerability of lacosamide (200, 400 and 600 mg/day given in two divided doses) in a total of over 1300 adults with uncontrolled focal seizures. Patients in these trials were taking at least one to three AEDs and many of the patients had previously tried at least seven AEDs. Across these studies significantly greater than 50% responder rates and reductions in median seizure frequency were seen versus placebo. Lacosamide was also generally well tolerated with the most common adverse events of lacosamide (>10% and greater than placebo) reported in these trials including dizziness, nausea, diplopia and headache.[61]

Lacosamide selectively enhances slow inactivation of voltage-gated sodium channels, resulting in stabilisation of hyperexcitable physiological neuronal excitability (Figure 1.1). In addition, it may bind with collapsin response mediator protein-2 (CRMP-2), a protein mainly expressed in the central nervous system and involved in neuronal differentiation and axonal outgrowth.[61]

The evidence so far is that lacosamide has proven efficacy and long retention rates in difficult to treat patients.[61] It is particularly important in adjunctive AED therapy because of minimal drug to drug interactions, good safety and tolerability, parenteral formulations and novel mechanism/s of action different than any other AED co-medication.[61]

Eslicarbazepine (Exalief® and Zebinix®) acetate, a derivative of carbamazepine, is the second AED licensed this year (April 2009) by the EMEA (it is not yet approved by FDA) as adjunctive therapy in adults ($\geq$ 18 years of age) with focal seizures with or without secondarily GTCS. It was developed with the intention to have no auto-induction and less interaction potential with other drugs than its parent drug carbamazepine by preventing the formation of toxic epoxide metabolites such as carbamazepine-10,11 epoxide. However, this promise does not appear to have been fulfilled because eslicarbazepine acetate is associated with significant interactions with drugs eliminated by metabolism through CYP3A4 (carbamazepine, phenytoin, phenobarbital, topiramate) or conjugation through the UDP-glucuronyltransferases (lamotrigine) and with oral hormonal contraception. Such interactions make the use of an AED problematic in adjunctive therapy and particularly when taken concomitantly with drugs of the same mechanism of action (carbamazepine, lamotrigine, phenytoin). Of benefit is that the rate of rash (1.1%) and hyponatraemia (less than 1%) with eslicarbazepine acetate is less than with carbamazepine and oxcarbazepine.

Newly diagnosed epilepsy

'Newly diagnosed epilepsy' (or newly identified epilepsy) is a general term for encompassing all types of epilepsy that are newly identified and firmly diagnosed by physicians irrespective of cause and prognosis. It includes any patient of any age with any form of seizure who seeks medical attention for the first time because of paroxysmal events that are diagnosed as epileptic seizures. Newly diagnosed epilepsy is not a diagnostic or therapeutic entity. Its purpose should be to emphasise that these patients require meticulous medical support with regard to diagnosis and treatment, which is thoroughly demanding. At this stage of first confirmation of diagnosis, medical decisions may affect the rest of the patient's life and often the lives of their families. Social and psychological support for the impact that such a diagnosis may have is a significant aspect of proper management. AED efficacy and ADRs are not determined by how long before the onset of treatment a diagnosis of seizures has been established.

'Newly diagnosed epilepsy' is not synonymous with 'new-onset epilepsy' with which it is incorrectly equated. Many patients have onset of seizures several years before seeking medical attention.

The management of patients with newly diagnosed epilepsy demands a precise diagnosis of both seizures and syndrome. Unifying them as a single therapeutic category[62] discourages diagnostic precision and encourages the use of inappropriate AED trial strategies (see Table 1.1).

Starting AED treatment in newly diagnosed epilepsy

The decision to start AED treatment needs to be thoroughly considered. It should not be a knee-jerk reaction to a crisis about a dramatic convulsive event that may not even be an epileptic seizure. Starting an AED often implies continuous daily medication for many years, which is sometimes life-long. Therefore, this should be strictly initiated in those with an unacceptably high rate of seizure recurrence or high risk of seizure injury. Some patients do not need prophylactic treatment, as in febrile and benign childhood focal seizures. In others the avoidance of precipitating factors may be sufficiently prophylactic, as in some reflex seizures or in individuals with a low threshold to seizures. For those in need of prophylactic treatment, the first-choice AED should primarily be in accordance with the seizure type (Table 1.1). AEDs beneficial for focal epilepsy may be detrimental for IGEs (Table 1.1). Even among IGEs, an AED beneficial in one type may be ineffective or aggravate another seizure type (Table 1.1).

Before starting prophylactic anti-epileptic medication in a patient with newly diagnosed seizures, a physician should be confident of the following:

1. *The patient unequivocally has epileptic seizures.*
 This requires definite exclusion of any imitators of epileptic seizures.
2. *The epileptic seizures of the patient need treatment.*
 This requires precise diagnosis of the epileptic syndrome and the type of seizures, their frequency and severity, their likelihood of relapse or remission, precipitating factors and the patient/family concerns and understanding of the risks versus benefits of the AED. Hard and fast rules are not always applicable.
3. *The most appropriate AED is selected for this particular patient with this particular type of seizure(s).*

The appropriate AED is that which is the most likely of all others to be truly prophylactic as monotherapy (single-drug treatment) for the seizures of the patient without causing undue ADRs (Tables 1.1 and 1.2). Carefully consider and exclude AEDs that may worsen or be ineffective in this particular type of seizures.

An AED is contraindicated not only when it exaggerates seizures, but also when it is ineffective in controlling the seizures that it is supposed to treat. It may cause unnecessary ADRs and deprive the patient of the therapeutic effect that could be provided by another appropriate AED.

4. *The starting dose and titration* of the selected drug should be in accordance with the appropriate recommendations, the age and, primarily, the particular needs of the treated patient.

All these should be thoroughly explained to the patient/guardian and it should be ensured that this is well understood.

The following should also be taken into consideration in deciding how to start and escalate the selected AED:

- patients, particularly with newly identified epilepsy, respond to their first-ever AED at low dosage and are prone to develop ADRs (biological, cognitive or behavioural), which in 15% of them lead to AED discontinuation
- some patients develop ADRs easily even at an AED dose below the minimal limit of the target (therapeutic) range, whereas others are resistant to AEDs even at the maximum limit of the target range
- even for patients with the same type of seizures and the same AED, seizure control may be achieved with a drug concentration below, within or above the target range.

Useful clinical notes

Steps from titration to maintenance AED dose

- Explain and give in writing the recommended dose to be used and the rate of escalation of the AED.
- Allow the patient to self-regulate the rate of dose and time escalation in terms of both the dose of and the time intervals for taking the AED.
- The first dose (test dose) should be taken at night before sleep. If ADRs cause significant discomfort the test dose should be decreased to half and tried again the next night.
- The patient should be at liberty to prolong the escalation time and reduce the escalation dose to suit his or her own reaction to the AED.
- Warn that any type of idiosyncratic reactions such as rash (even if mild) should be reported immediately so as to prevent more serious and sometimes life-threatening events.
- Clarify that minor ADRs such as fatigue or somnolence are usually dose related and should not discourage escalation unless they interfere with the patient's daily activities.
- If seizures are controlled at some stage during the escalation, this should be the maintenance dose (irrespective of whether this is smaller than the recommended dose).

Monotherapy

Patients should be treated with a single AED (monotherapy) because of better efficacy, minimisation of ADRs and drug interactions, and improved compliance. Monotherapy with an appropriately selected AED at an appropriate target dose achieves complete control of seizures in 50–70% of patients. In one study, almost half the newly diagnosed patients of any type (symptomatic or idiopathic) became seizure free on their first-ever AED, with more than 90% doing so at modest dosing.[63] If seizures continue, titrating to the limit of tolerability will achieve additional seizure control in about 20% of patients, but be aware of the increased risk of ADRs.

The selected AED should be considered as a failure if unacceptable ADRs occur, seizures continue or new treatment-emergent seizures appear. In any of these events, another AED that fulfils therapeutic expectations for success should be initiated. The first AED should be gradually withdrawn so as to re-establish monotherapy. Switching between AEDs must be carried out cautiously, slowly withdrawing the first drug only after the second drug has reached an adequate therapeutic dosage.

Important practical note

Non-compliance or failing to understand and follow the instructions for AED treatment is a major cause of therapeutic failure. This can often be improved with the use of AED-dispenser systems, which are widely available through pharmacies. These usually come in small boxes for a weekly or longer supply of each individual patient's tablets or capsules to be taken at the time and date shown. These are useful even for patients who comply well, but who often may be uncertain whether or not they have taken their medication.

Rational polytherapy

Polytherapy (combination, adjunctive or 'add-on' therapy) should be considered only when attempts at monotherapy with an AED have not resulted in freedom from seizures. If trials of combination therapy do not bring about worthwhile benefits, treatment should revert to the regimen (monotherapy or polytherapy) that has proved most acceptable to the patient in terms of providing the best balance between effectiveness in reducing seizure frequency and the tolerability of ADRs.

The risks of polytherapy include
- more ADRs
- frequent unwanted interactions with other drugs,
- an increased risk of teratogenicity,
- inability to evaluate the efficacy and ADRs of individual AED agents, and
- poor compliance.

However, polytherapy is infrequently more desirable than monotherapy; for example, in JME patients on valproate, adding small doses of clonazepam for continuing disturbing myoclonic jerks or small doses of lamotrigine for continuing serious absences may be more beneficial than increasing the dose of valproate.

Rational polytherapy is often needed for 30–50% of patients who are unsatisfactorily controlled with a single AED. This is much higher in patients with symptomatic focal epilepsies than in patients with IGEs. A recent study showed that the chance to become seizure free declines by 75% after every 3 lifetime used AEDs, leaving up to 16.6% of patients uncontrolled after failure of three previous AEDs.[64] Similarly, the chance to be a 50% responder also declines by 50% after every 2 lifetime used AEDs.[64] Almost all epileptic encephalopathies require polytherapy. Initially, a second drug is added to the agent, which showed better efficacy and tolerability in monotherapy. The choice of a second or sometimes a third drug depends on many factors such as efficacy, ADRs, interactions with other drugs, mode of action and the need for laboratory testing (Table 1.3).

The addition of an AED to other AEDs that have partially or totally failed or have made the situation worse is a formidable task for a physician, especially when faced with a disappointed and frustrated patient. Polytherapy with more than three drugs is discouraged because adverse reactions become more prominent, with little if any seizure improvement.

Polytherapy can be irrational and hazardous if a diagnosis is incorrect and AED indications/contraindications are violated.

The decision for polytherapy should first scrutinise the possible/probable reasons why the monotherapy failed. These should thoroughly examine the following possibilities, which often require re-evaluation of diagnosis (genuine epileptic seizures? what type of seizures?):

- the patient does not suffer from epileptic seizures
- the patient has both genuine epileptic and non-epileptic seizures
- the patient has focal and no generalised seizures or *vice versa*
- the AED used as monotherapy was not suitable for the particular type of seizures in this patient because of contraindications (tiagabine or carbamazepine in absences or myoclonic jerks, and lamotrigine in myoclonic epilepsies), weak efficacy (valproate or gabapentin in focal seizures) or total ineffectiveness (gabapentin in primarily GTCSs)
- non-compliance, which varies from unwillingness to take medication to occasionally forgetting or missing the AED dose; violation of particularly eminent seizure-precipitating factors such as photic stimulation, sleep deprivation and alcohol or drug abuse.

The ideal profile of an AED for polytherapeutic purposes includes all the factors that are important for monotherapy (Table 1.3), but with particular emphasis on the following points.

Strength of efficacy which may be increased or weakened by pharmacokinetic and pharmaco-dynamic interactions.

Safety and tolerability (Table 1.2), which are often worsened by pharmacokinetic and pharmacodynamic interactions.

Interactions with other AEDs, whether pharmacokinetic, pharmacodynamic or both, are particularly unwanted in polytherapy (Tables 1.6 and 1.7). Raising the levels of concomitant AEDs and pharmacodynamic interactions may lead to toxic effects. Conversely, decreasing their levels may increase and worsen seizures causing a vicious cycle in clinical management. With the exception of lacosamide, levetiracetam and gabapentin, all other newer AEDs exhibit sometimes complex, undesirable, drug–drug interactions. Of the newer AEDs, lamotrigine is probably the worst of all. Lamotrigine:

- requires different dosage and titration schemes when combined with hepatic enzyme inducers and when combined with valproate
- pharmacodynamic interactions enhance toxicity and teratogenicity (although pharmacodynamic interactions have a beneficial effect on efficacy)
- its levels lower more than half during pregnancy or hormonal contraception.

Different mechanisms of action in relation to other concurrent AEDs (Table 1.8). Anti-epileptic drug–drug interactions may be purely additive, antagonistic or synergistic. AEDs with the same mechanism of action would be expected to be additive, while combining AEDs with different mechanisms of action may have synergistic effects.[65] A sodium channel blocker AED combined with another that increases the GABA-ergic neurotransmission or that has multiple mechanisms is generally more effective than a combination of two sodium channel blockers.[66] An AED is unlikely to have better success and more likely to have additive ADRs if added to another AED with the same mechanism of action.[66] Lacosamide and levetiracetam appear to have novel modes of action.[61,67]

Converting from polytherapy to monotherapy

Evidence from studies with older and newer AEDs shows that a significant number of patients can be converted successfully from polytherapy to monotherapy without losing seizure control and, in some cases, with improved seizure control. In these cases the AED that appears, after careful consideration, to be the least effective is gradually withdrawn. 'Gradually' sometimes means in steps of weeks or months. This should be particularly slow for certain AEDs, such as phenobarbital and benzodiazepines, in order to avoid withdrawal seizures.

Total AED withdrawal

Consideration of total withdrawal of AEDs is needed in the following patients:

- patients who do not suffer from epileptic seizures
- patients suffering from age-related and age-limited epileptic syndromes who have reached an appropriate age of remission

- patients who are seizure free for more than 3–5 years, provided that they do not suffer from epileptic syndromes requiring long-term treatment such as JME.

Discontinuation of AEDs should be extremely slow, in small doses and in long steps of weeks or months. The rate of relapse increases with a faster rate of AED discontinuation. Furthermore, with fast discontinuation of AEDs there is a risk of seizures that are directly related to the withdrawal effects of certain AEDs (phenobarbital and benzodiazepines).

Before AED withdrawal, there is a need for a thorough re-evaluation of the patient. The presence of even minor and infrequent seizures specifies active disease. Conversely, the occurrence of such seizures in the process of AED discontinuation mandates restoration of AED medication.

Over-medication in terms of the number of AEDs and doses and length of exposure is undesirable but common. Treatment should be reviewed at regular intervals to ensure that patients are not maintained for long periods on drugs that are ineffective, poorly tolerated or not needed, and that concordance with prescribed medication is maintained.

A normal EEG does not mean that AED withdrawal is safe. Conversely, ictal EEG abnormalities associated with clinical manifestations (e.g. jerks or absences) is a definite indicator for continuing proper AED treatment.

Generic versus brand or generic to generic AED prescribing

A patient who is stabilised with an AED in terms of seizure control and minimal ADRs should remain in the same brand or the particular generic product, which are not interchangeable without risks.

When an AED is first prescribed, this can be a brand or a generic product providing that the latter has been truly tested in regard to the credibility of its manufacturers and bioequivalence with the brand product. Titration and maintenance should be with the same AED product.

It is unreasonable to switch from one to another AED, either from an expensive branded AED to a cheaper bioequivalent generic product or vice versa. It is unnecessary and may impose significant risk to the patient.

When such substitution is attempted the patient should be well informed of possible consequences, such as seizure relapse or ADRs.

Prescriptions should clearly indicate the type of AED formulation to be used even for generic products.

AEDs are first licensed and used with their brand name and this is protected by granted patents and exclusivity. Patents are granted anywhere along the development lifeline of a drug and can encompass a wide range of claims. Exclusivity is a term describing marketing rights granted upon approval of a drug and can run concurrently with a patent or not. Exclusivity was designed to promote a balance between new drug innovation and generic drug competition. Generic AEDs are usually introduced after patents and exclusivity have been expired with the single aim to reduce the cost of the medication.

There is considerable concern amongst physicians and patients about the efficacy and safety of brand to generic AED substitution or vice versa and also from one to another generic drug of different manufacturers.[68–76]

These concerns have been reasonably raised because of well documented breakthrough seizures, emergency treated epilepsy-events and toxicity as a result of such substitutions. These unwanted and preventable adverse effects are well documented from the time of Epanutin® to phenytoin[77] and Mysoline® to primidone substitutions.

Substitution from one to another AED of the same active substance is safe only when these are of therapeutic equivalence: "Drug products are considered to be therapeutic equivalents ... if they can be expected to have the same clinical effect and safety profile when administered to patients under the conditions specified in the labeling." However, even when the generic product is from a reliable source (something that is beyond the role of prescribing physicians) there may be problems with their therapeutic equivalence particularly in terms of bioavailability and pharmacokinetic profiles.

AEDs are particularly vulnerable in these changes, because most have a narrow reference concentration index between drug levels that are therapeutic and those that may cause ADRs.

It is because of these problems that formal recommendations worldwide uniformly warn against such substitutions of AEDs (see citations in reference):[69]

"Changing the formulation or brand of any AED is not recommended because different preparations may vary in bioavailability or have different pharmacokinetic profiles and, thus, increased potential for reduced effect or excessive side-effects." (National Institute for Health and Clinical Excellence-UK).[2]

"For AEDs, small variations in concentrations between name-brands and their generic equivalents can cause toxic effects and/or seizures when taken by patients with epilepsy. The AAN believes that the authorities should give complete physician autonomy in prescribing AEDs." (American Academy of Neurology).[75]

In regard to the implications of changing AED formulations for TDM the recent ILAE position paper recommends:[78]

(a) When an AED formulation is changed, e.g., when switching to/from generic formulations, measuring the plasma concentration of the AED before and after the change may help in identifying potential alterations in steady-state drug concentrations resulting from differences in bioavailability.

(b) When patients are switched to a formulation with modified-release characteristics (for example, from an immediate-release to a sustained-release formulations), or when dosing schedule is changed (for example, from twice daily to once daily administration), interpretation of TDM data should also take into account the expected variation in diurnal drug concentration profile. In some instances, collection of two or more blood samples at different intervals after drug intake may be desirable to fully assess the concentration profile change.

Evidence for AED treatment recommendations in clinical practice

In clinical practice a physician faces a colossal task not only to make the correct diagnosis for a patient but also to correctly identify which is the best AED option for both the patient and their particular type of seizure and syndrome. However, such judgement requires huge, extensive, continually updated and multilevel knowledge, which even expert clinical epileptologists may not have. Therefore, it is fundamental for physicians to be informed about the best existing evidence for AED treatment in clinical practice.

> *Clinicians need advice – they always have, but with the multiplicity of therapies now available, this need is pressing.*[79]

Recommendations and guidelines should be clear for each AED: what priority and for what type of seizures they are effective, potentially useful, ineffective, contraindicated or harmful. Ideally, these recommendations should be based on unequivocal documentation but often this is limited to probable, possible or purely anecdotal evidence.

Evidence-based recommendations

Evidence-based medicine (EBM),[80,81] which was introduced in 1991, is a welcome healthcare practice that is based on integrating the knowledge gained from the best available research evidence and clinical expertise with patients' values and circumstances.

EBM is defined as 'the conscientious, explicit, and judicious use of current best evidence in making decisions about the care of individual patients' and the practice of EBM means 'integrating individual clinical expertise with the best available external clinical evidence from systematic research'.[80]

In therapy, EBM aims to treat patients according to the best available evidence and its purpose is to protect patients from treatments based on untested ideas. The way to test which treatment is best is usually by appropriate RCTs, which are typically double-blind. In many instances when solid evidence is lacking or not directly applicable to a given patient, EBM endorses lower levels of evidence (e.g. ongoing importance of fundamental clinical skills, sound clinical reasoning, accumulated experience and common sense).

Problems with RCTs include:

- bad quality; the Consolidated Standards for Reporting of Trials (CONSERT) statement was developed in an attempt to combat this problem

- designs for regulatory purposes and of no clinical relevance
- their high cost, which often makes RCTs unapproachable or limited
- their misuse by special interest groups.[81]

Approximately a fifth of drugs approved by regulatory authorities are subsequently withdrawn due to post-marketing evidence of imposing health risk.

The results of EBM often clash with the agenda of special interest groups... We need to alert clinicians and patients to studies showing that reviews sponsored by the industry almost always favour the sponsor's product, whereas those that aren't sponsored by such companies do not. We also need to provide patients and the general public with the tools to enable them to understand and evaluate systematic reviews.[81]

The problems with RCTs in epilepsies are similar to those of other treatments and I quote protagonists of RCTs:

These studies are almost always sponsored by the pharmaceutical company that manufactures the newer drug, and almost always conclude that the newer drug is equally as effective but better tolerated than the established drug.[82]

Unfortunately, methodological problems, including small sample size, questionable selection of patients, titration schedules, dose and dose form, and short duration of study, have limited the acceptance of the results.[82]

Rating classification schemes for RCTs have the sole purpose of eliminating bias in studies. They do not address whether the study results are clinically valid.[83]

Results were potentially confounded by errors in seizure classification and failure to measure seizures other than tonic clonic during follow-up.[84]

Misclassification of patients may have confounded the results... The age distribution of adults classified as having generalized seizures indicated that significant numbers of patients may have had their seizures misclassified.[85]

Diagnostic uncertainties and methodological pressures confound the analysis of these studies.

The school of clinical epileptology that I follow may find some RCTs unacceptable both in their methodology and in their proposals on the use of AEDs in clinical practice for the principal reason that they examine AED response in a unified definition of 'epilepsy' irrespective of the type of epileptic seizures or patient group. Children's epilepsies and management differ from adults in many respects. Women of childbearing age mandate a different approach.

One RCT[62] promotes the detrimental, indiscriminate use of carbamazepine and valproate because 'neither of them is regarded as the single drug of choice for all patients with newly diagnosed epilepsy'[62] despite established documentation that these are two different AEDs with different indications and contraindications in partial and generalised epilepsies.

Another, more recent RCT unifies *all* patients (normal or neurodevelopmentally impaired children, women, men and elderly) with *all* types of seizures. The physician's intention to treat with carbamazepine or valproate is the only differentiating question in the quest of what is the best AED treatment.[84]

We have also seen some disasters. Numerous RCTs showed that vigabatrin was a relatively safe drug with a relatively benign adverse-effect profile. A RCT in 1999 found vigabatrin 'less effective but better tolerated than carbamazepine in patients with partial epilepsies'.[86] This was 2 years after the first report of vigabatrin-emergent irreversible peripheral visual field defects,[87] which occur in 40% of the patients receiving vigabatrin and ended its use in epilepsies other than the West syndrome.

These issues with RCTs may compromise purely evidence-based recommendations[88] and for multiple reasons there are significant difficulties in extrapolating data from RCTs to clinical practice.[89] This is well reflected in the discrepancies between guidelines derived from the same data.[79,90] Partly as a result, such influential recommendations may mislead physicians in the appropriate use of newer AEDs and inadvertently perpetuate suboptimal practice in new clinical trials.

> One striking result of the increasing plethora of guidelines is the apparent paradox that recommendations differ from one guideline to another, although each usually purports to use the same evidence base and to exhibit scientific objectivity.[79]

Furthermore, in some of these formal recommendations there is a conspicuous bias in favour of the newer AEDs. A formal guideline emphasises that:

> The older AEDs as a class have complex pharmacokinetics. Four of the six AEDs available prior to 1990 (phenytoin, carbamazepine, phenobarbital and primidone) are hepatic enzyme inducers. Induction not only complicates combination AED therapy but also changes internal hormonal milieu in possibly important ways. Intrinsic compounds, such as sex steroids and vitamin D, are hypermetabolised. This can lead to reproductive dysfunction and osteopenia. Enzyme-inducing AEDs produce important interactions with many commonly used medications, such as warfarin, oral contraceptives, calcium channel antagonists and chemotherapeutic agents, to name a few. Valproate, in contrast, is a potent hepatic inhibitor. There is controversy about the impact of valproate on the hormonal milieu and inhibition leads to important drug interactions with AEDs as well as other classes. The newer agents are involved in many fewer drug interactions. Many of the newer agents have little if any effect on the CYP450 enzyme system and other metabolic pathways.[91]

However, such a generalisation, although correct if older and newer AEDs are considered as two different 'classes', is inadequate without specifying that certain newer AEDs have similar or even worse drug–drug interactions in comparison with certain older AEDs. Newer AEDs are not innocent. All newer AEDs but levetiracetam (characterised as ideal),[92,93] lacosamide, pregabalin, and gabapentin sometimes exhibit complex undesirable drug–drug interactions.

A recent editorial by Simon Shorvon in *Epilepsia* – *We live in the age of the clinical guideline* – should be read by all physicians.[79] It is the most objective, wise and brave paper published on these important issues as evident by the following extracts[79] with which I fully agree:

> *An avalanche of guidelines risks burying the clinician in a white snow of double-talk and humbug, and is not wholly in the best interests either of medicine or of patients.*

> *Political interference, personal ego and prejudice are common in guideline committees.*

> *Commercially funded systematic reviews are prone to bias in favour of the sponsor and have been shown to score badly on scientific validity.*

> *Other inherent limitations further reduce the practical value of clinical guidelines. One (obvious) issue is the fact that knowledge advances: time is no friend to the clinical guideline.*

> *The blanket advice of many restrictive guidelines, based on a limited number of RCTs that are narrow in their scope, almost invariably ignores the fact that optimal therapy can differ in different syndromes and in different clinical settings.*

On medicolegal aspects Shorvon also emphasises:[79]

> *Guidelines are not regulations but often are treated as such.*

> *Tailoring therapy to individual patients, whether within or outwith a guideline recommendation, remains a prerogative that doctors should not sacrifice.*

Poverty of reliable RCTs in epilepsies

The 2006 ILAE report[44] is the most authoritative evidence-based review and analysis of the efficacy and effectiveness of AEDs as initial monotherapy for epileptic seizures, although myoclonic seizures have not been assessed. It also reviews evidence-based AED efficacy and effectiveness as initial monotherapy in JME, childhood absence epilepsy and rolandic epilepsy. The analysis applied a rating scale of evidence of class I (best) to class IV (worst) to potentially relevant reports from 1940 until July 2005. The level of evidence for the conclusions was also graded from A (a high degree of reliability) to F (a low degree of reliability).

The ILAE report concluded that:

It is clear that an alarming lack of well-designed, properly conducted epilepsy RCTs exist... the absence of rigorous comprehensive adverse effects data makes it impossible to develop an evidence-based guideline aimed at identifying the overall optimal recommended initial monotherapy AED. There is an especially alarming lack of well-designed, properly conducted RCTs for patients with generalized seizures/epilepsies and for children in general. The majority of relevant existing RCTs have significant methodologic problems that limit their applicability to this guideline's clinically relevant main question.[44]

The following recommendations were made:

Multicenter, multinational efforts are needed to design, conduct and analyze future clinically relevant RCTs that can answer the many outstanding questions identified in this guideline. The ultimate choice of an AED for any individual patient with newly diagnosed or untreated epilepsy should include consideration of the strength of the efficacy and effectiveness evidence for each AED along with other variables such as the AED safety and tolerability profile, pharmacokinetic properties, formulations, and expense. When selecting a patient's AED, physicians and patients should consider all relevant variables and not just efficacy and effectiveness.[44]

Based on available efficacy and effectiveness evidence alone and only for RCTs published before July 2005, recommendations at levels A and B were possible for:

- adults with newly diagnosed or untreated focal seizures: carbamazepine (A), phenytoin (A) and valproate (B)
- children with newly diagnosed or untreated focal seizures: oxcarbazepine (A)
- elderly with newly diagnosed or untreated focal seizures: lamotrigine (A) and gabapentin (A)
- adults with GTCSs: none has reached level A or B
- children with GTCSs: none has reached level A or B
- children with absence seizures: none has reached level A or B
- rolandic epilepsy: none has reached level A or B
- JME: none has reached level A or B.

Note

Levetiracetam has not been considered in the above recommendation because the relevant RCT of Brodie *et al*[94] has only recently been published. The results of this class 1 with A level of evidence RCT earned levetiracetam approval as a first-line monotherapy in the treatment of focal epilepsy.

Evidence-based recommendations in this book

The recommendations made in this book are based on a thorough review of the efficacy, tolerability, safety and interactions, and other essential parameters involved in the choice of AEDs (Tables 1.3 and 1.12). The following sources were used:

- evidence-based reports, RCTs, reviews and expert assessments and guidelines of AED treatment in children and adults
- post-marketing open studies, and observational and case reports that appeared in full papers or abstract forms
- expert physicians' experiences of the clinical use of AEDs, which were obtained through critical discussions or personal correspondence with them
- pathophysiology of seizures and mechanisms of actions in animal models as supportive rather than conclusive evidence of clinical usefulness.

It is reassuring that important conclusions made in my previous publications proved to be correct, in particular with respect to the following recommendations:

- valproate is the superior AED for generalised epilepsies but its use as monotherapy in focal epilepsies is unwise
- vigabatrin and tiagabine are pro-absence AEDs that induce rather than treat absence epilepsies
- gabapentin has the least efficacy of the newer AEDs in focal epilepsies and is ineffective in IGEs
- pregabalin does not appear to have a promising profile as an AED
- lamotrigine may not be appropriate for monotherapy in JME (it may aggravate myoclonic jerks), where its beneficial effect is mainly seen when combined with valproate
- levetiracetam is a very effective broad-spectrum newer AED in focal[94] and generalised[95] epilepsies; it is the only one of the newer AEDs licensed for myoclonic seizures of JME.

Therapeutic drug monitoring

Therapeutic drug monitoring (TDM), in which plasma concentrations of AEDs are measured, can have a valuable role in guiding patient management provided that concentrations are measured with a clear indication and are interpreted critically, taking into account the whole clinical context.[78]

Useful recommendation

The recent ILAE position paper of 2008[78] is a practice guideline for TDM and is highly recommended for further reading and citations. It also provides pharmacokinetic details, interactions with other AEDs, and reference ranges for each AED and discusses the role of TDM in children and the elderly and during pregnancy.

Reference ranges which laboratories can quote and which clinicians can use as a guide are not synonymous with therapeutic ranges.[78]

Pragmatic recommendations for AED treatment with older and newer AEDs for epileptic seizures and main epileptic syndromes

Seizures/syndromes	First-line AEDs* (in order of priority)	Second-line AEDs* (in order of priority)
Focal (simple and complex) seizures with or without secondarily GTCSs	Carbamazepine, phenytoin, phenobarbital *Levetiracetam, oxcarbazepine, lamotrigine, topiramate*	Clobazam, valproate, *Lacosamide, gabapentin, zonisamide, pregabalin, tiagabine*
Primarily GTCSs only	Valproate, phenobarbital, phenytoin *Levetiracetam, lamotrigine, topiramate*	Carbamazepine *Oxcarbazepine*
Myoclonic seizures only	Clonazepam, valproate, phenobarbital *Levetiracetam*	Phenytoin, ethosuximide *Topiramate, zonisamide*
Absence seizures only(typical and atypical)	Valproate, ethosuximide *Lamotrigine*	Clonazepam *Levetiracetam, zonisamide, topiramate*
Negative myoclonic andatonic seizures	Ethosuxide, valproate *Levetiracetam*	Clonazepam *Zonisamide, topiramate*
Tonic seizures	Valproate, phenytoin, phenobarbital *Topiramate, lamotrigine*	Clonazepam, clobazam *Zonisamide*
Benign childhood focal seizures and syndromes	Carbamazepine, valproate, sulthiame, clobazam *Levetiracetam, oxcarbazepine, lamotrigine*	*Gabapentin, lacosamide, zonisamide*
All symptomatic and cryptogenic syndromes of focal epilepsies	Carbamazepine, phenytoin, phenobarbital *Levetiracetam, oxcarbazepine, lamotrigine, topiramate*	Clobazam, valproate *Lacosamide, gabapentin, zonisamide, pregabalin, tiagabine*
Childhood absence epilepsy	Ethosuxide, valproate *Lamotrigine*	Clonazepam
Juvenile absence epilepsy	Valproate, ethosuximide *Lamotrigine*	Clonazepam *Levetiracetam, zonisamide, topiramate*
Juvenile myoclonic epilepsy	Valproate, phenobarbital *Levetiracetam, topiramate*	Clonazepam, ethosuximide *Zonisamide, lamotrigine*
Photosensitive andother reflex seizures	Valproate *Levetiracetam*	Clonazepam *Lamotrigine*
Lennox–Gastaut syndrome and other epileptic encephalopathies (AEDs largely depend on predominant seizure type)	Valproate *Lamotrigine, levetiracetam, rufinamide, topiramide, zonisamide*	Clobazam, clonazepam, ethosuximide, phenytoin *Felbamate, stiripentol (Dravet syndrome only)*

Table 1.12 *Older AEDs are shown in roman; newer AEDs are shown in blue italics. The table is only indicative of AEDs to use in each of the epileptic seizures or syndromes. Priority depends on AED properties, whether monotherapy or polytherapy is used, and the needs of individual patients, as detailed in this book. In choosing an AED from this table, the order of priority is between the first in the list of older or newer AEDs in the middle column.

The "reference range" of an AED is a statistical standard of the AED concentration. It is derived from population studies and indicates the level at which most patients achieve optimal seizure control. It specifies a lower limit below which a therapeutic response is relatively unlikely to occur, and an upper limit above which toxicity is relatively likely to occur.[78,95] Concentrations lying within the reference range are not "normal" because the "normal" concentration of a drug in a living organism is zero.

> *Reference range is the optimal drug concentration range at which most patients achieve the desired therapeutic effect with no undesirable side effects.*

Reference range is a useful guideline, but effective AED maintenance dosing should be based mainly on clinical criteria because the inter-patient variability is considerable. Many patients can achieve therapeutic benefit at plasma drug concentrations outside these ranges. Some patients are well controlled below the low range-limit, whereas others achieve seizure freedom above the upper range-limit. Some patients are free of adverse reactions even at 'toxic' target levels, whereas others may develop adverse reactions that are unacceptable for them at trough levels, which are just measurable. Thus, concentrations lying within the reference range may not necessarily be "therapeutic", "effective", or "optimal" and therefore it is recommended that these adjectives not be used when reporting the results.[78] The correct reporting terminology should be "The result lies within/above/below the reference range".[78] It is because of these reasons that the term therapeutic range has been introduced.

The "therapeutic range" is defined as the range of drug concentrations that is associated with the best achievable response in a given person, and therefore can only be determined for the specific individual.

Plasma and saliva TDM

Serum or plasma represents the matrix of choice for TDM, and although they can be used interchangeably it is preferable to use one or the other.[78] Saliva is a matrix of increasing utility, but only for some AEDs.

Useful practical note

TDM: rule of thumb for individual patients

The level is 'therapeutic' when, and only when, the patient is free of seizures and free of ADRs regardless of numbers in TDM. The dose of an AED is adequate if seizures are controlled and if ADRs are not present or these are mild. The dose is high if intolerable adverse reactions are present irrespective of seizure control.

Routine TDM measures the total (free and protein-bound) plasma concentration of an AED in a blood sample. The values provided do not discriminate between the amount of the protein bound drug and that which is free (unbound) and pharmacologically active.[78] Thus, monitoring free plasma concentrations is useful in clinical settings when protein binding is altered, such as in hypoalbuminemia (e.g. in pregnancy, in old age, and in liver disease, renal disease, and many other pathological conditions), in conditions associated with accumulation of endogenous displacing agents (e.g., uraemia), and following administration of drugs which compete for plasma protein binding sites. Phenytoin and valproate are highly protein-bound and consequently susceptible to variable binding.

Saliva TDM is rarely used in clinical practice because samples are often contaminated in the mouth, thereby making the results unreliable. Advantages of saliva TDM of AEDs as an alternative to plasma TDM include:

- collection is simple and non-invasive
- it can be especially useful in patients with disabilities and is preferred by children and their parents
- for most AEDs, measured concentrations reflect the free (pharmacologically relevant) concentration in blood.

Disadvantages of saliva TDM include:

- the difficulty in measuring concentrations that may be lower than total plasma concentration
- the possibility of contamination and unreliable results due to the presence of drug residues in the mouth or leakage of drug-rich exudate, particularly in patients with gingivitis. To minimise contamination from drug residues, saliva sampling is best done before the next dose and after a good wash of the mouth

AEDs for which there are substantial data suggesting useful correlations between saliva concentrations and free plasma concentrations include carbamazepine, ethosuximide, gabapentin, lamotrigine, levetiracetam, oxcarbazepine, phenytoin, primidone, topiramate, and vigabatrin. For drugs with pK values close to physiological pH (e.g., valproate and phenobarbital), salivary concentrations can be highly variable or erratic; saliva TDM should not be used for these drugs.

Clinical applications

Monitoring the plasma levels of AEDs is useful in clinical practice for maximising seizure control and minimising adverse reactions, provided that it is selectively and appropriately used in response to a patient-specific pharmacokinetic or pharmacodynamic issue or problem.[78,97,98]

Of the older AEDs, phenytoin, phenobarbital and carbamazepine are more likely to necessitate TDM; valproate has a number of peculiarities and variability. The usefulness of TDM has been initially questioned for most of the newer AEDs because a wide range of plasma concentrations are associated with clinical efficacy and no useful or considerable overlap is reported between 'concentration–effect' and 'concentration–toxicity'. This view has been recently revised, particularly in women, because plasma concentrations of some newer AEDs are significantly influenced by hormonal contraception and pregnancy (see forthcoming section of the management of women with epilepsy). In co-medication also enzyme-inducers significantly affect plasma levels of lamotrigine and topiramate levels.[99]

Current tentative reference ranges for each of the newer AEDs have been reported and these are stated in the pharmacopoeia and in references.[78,94,100]

Solid evidence for the usefulness of TDM in improving clinical outcome is scarce and debated.[78,101]

In clinical practice TDM is recommended:[78,100]

- for establishing 'baseline' effective concentrations (therapeutic range) in patients who have been successfully stabilised, enabling future comparisons to assess potential causes for a change in drug response, for example if seizures recur, in pregnancy or in patients in need of polytherapy or other medications
- for evaluating potential causes for lack or loss of efficacy
- for evaluating potential causes for toxicity
- to assess compliance, particularly in patients with uncontrolled seizures or breakthrough seizures
- to guide dosage adjustment in situations associated with increased pharmacokinetic variability (e.g., children, the elderly, patients with associated diseases, drug formulation changes) when a potentially important pharmacokinetic change is anticipated (e.g., in pregnancy, or when an interacting drug is added or removed)
- to guide dose adjustments for AEDs with dose-dependent pharmacokinetics, particularly phenytoin.

TDM is complicated in polytherapy because it is unlikely that the reference range is the same when an AED is taken alone or in combination with other AEDs; for example, the toxicity from carbamazepine or valproate appears at higher plasma levels when these AEDs are used in monotherapy than when they are used in combination.

Useful clinical note

Regularly repeating TDM in patients who are controlled and with no sign of adverse reactions 'just to make sure that everything is ok' is totally discouraged.

Trough AED plasma levels are important with regard to efficacy, whereas peak AED plasma levels are important with regard to toxicity.

In treatment with carbamazepine or oxcarbazepine, diplopia is a sign of exceeding the drug dosage, irrespective of TDM levels.

Time of sampling

Sampling time and a meticulous dosage history is imperative for proper TDM utility in clinical practice.[78]

Sampling should be done at steady state, which occurs at 4–5 half-lives after starting treatment or a dose change. Half-life values and other pharmacokinetic parameters of AEDs can be found in the recent ILAE position paper.[78] Patient noncompliance within a period of 3–4 half-lives before the blood sample is drawn can significantly affect the plasma concentration and cause misinterpretation of the result. Plasma concentration may be underestimated when blood sampling is taken before a drug steady-state plasma is reached. Conversely, it may be overestimated when blood sampling is taken before auto-induction of carbamazepine is complete.[78]

For AEDs with a long half-life (e.g. ethosuximide, phenobarbital, phenytoin) timing is not important because fluctuations in plasma concentration are negligible in the course of a day; samples can be collected at any time.

For AEDs with a short half-life (e.g. carbamazepine, gabapentin, lamotrigine, levetiracetam, pregabalin, topiramate, valproate) it is important to standardise sampling time in relation to dose. For these AEDs it is recommended that blood samples are obtained before the first dose when the concentration is at its trough (which is useful for assessing ineffectiveness) and/or at a time of expected peak concentrations (which is useful for assessing toxicity).

Useful clinical note

There is no point to attempt TDM before a time interval of 4–5 half-lives of starting treatment or a dose change.

TDM is useful for assessing ineffectiveness when the AED plasma concentration is at its trough (before the next dose)

TDM is useful for assessing toxicity at times of expected peak concentrations

Considerations of adverse anti-epileptic drug reactions in the treatment of epilepsies

Adverse drug reactions (Table 1.2) should be thoroughly sought in patients treated with AEDs. Despite their significance, identifying ADRs is often neglected because of time constraints, confounding factors and the multiplicity of potential symptoms. Patients may also be reluctant to report them or they may confuse them with a consequence of their illness.

ADRs may be minor or severe, transient or progressive, reversible or irrevesrible, known, unknown or suspected. They vary significantly between AEDs and with dose, length of exposure, individual susceptibility, age, sex and comorbitidies. Emphasis is given to ADRs associated with use of older AEDs, though ADRs may also be highly significant with the use of newer AEDs. They are more likely to occur with polytherapy than monotherapy.

Patients, particularly with newly identified epilepsy, are prone to develop ADRs (biological, cognitive or behavioural), which in 15% of cases lead to AED discontinuation. Some patients develop ADRs readily even at an AED

dose below the minimal limit of the reference (therapeutic) range, while others
are resistant to ADRs even at the maximum limit of that range.

ADRs may be very common ($\geq 1/10$ per patient exposed to an AED), common
($\geq 1/100$ to $<1/10$) or uncommon ($\geq 1/1000$ to $<1/100$).

ADR associated with each AEDs and their particular effects in children, women
and elderly are frequently emphasised in this book.

Life-threatening ADRs

These are the most dreadful of all ADRs and carry a black box warning in their
package inserts.

Anticonvulsant hypersensitivity syndrome (AHS), though rare, is the most common
potentially fatal ADR linked with AEDs, occurring at a rate of 1000–10000
exposures.[102-109] Carbamazepine, felbamate, lamotrigine, oxcarbazepine,
phenytoin, phenobarbital and zonisamide are associated with frequent idiosyncratic
reactions and anticonvulsant hypersensitivity syndrome (AHS). The main clinical
manifestations of AHS consist of skin rashes, fever, tender lymphadenopathy,
eosinophilia, and hepatic and other systemic organ involvement. Diagnosis is
primarily based on the recognition of clinical symptoms.

The appearance of a rash is an early indicator that mandates the immediate
discontinuation of the responsible agent because it may progress to AHS and
Stevens–Johnson syndrome.

The underlying mechanisms of AHS are thought to have at least three
components: (a) deficiency or abnormality of the epoxide hydroxylase enzyme
that detoxifies the metabolites of aromatic amine AEDs, (b) reactivation of
herpes-type viruses, and (c) ethnic predisposition with certain human leukocyte
antigen subtypes.[103] To reflect recent advances in pharmacogenetics, the FDA
has issued an alarm on dangerous or even fatal skin reactions (Stevens Johnson
syndrome and toxic epidermal necrolysis) that can be caused by carbamazepine,
which are significantly more common in patients with the leukocyte antigen
subtype HLA-B*1502. This particular human leukocyte antigen allele occurs
almost exclusively in patients with ancestry across broad areas of Asia, including
South Asian Indians.   Genetic tests for HLA-B*1502 are already available.

There is usually a high degree (40–80%) of cross-sensitivity for AHS between
AEDs. Thus, patients with a history of AHS should avoid use of AEDs which have
the potential to cause AHS. Also, there is an increased risk of AHS amongst family
members of patients with AHS. AHS is nore common in children than adults.

AEDs that are unlikely to cause AHS are benzodiazepines, levetiracetam and
valproate (but the latter has been associated with increasing the AHS risk of
lamotrigine).[9]

Other life-threatening ADRs to AEDs and their preferential occurrence in age
groups or women are detailed in the description of each one of the AEDs and
the relevant sections. These include valproate-related hepatic and pancreatic
failure in young children, topiramate and zonisamide-related anhidosis and

so forth. Little is known about the cardiac ADRs of AEDs though these may also be potentially fatal, particularly in elderly and patients with pre-existing cardiological abnormalities.

Suicidal ideation that may lead to suicide has also attracted significant attention recently with another alert issued by FDA[111]. This was based on pooled analyses of 199 clinical trials of eleven AEDs (carbamazepine, felbamate, gabapentin, lamotrigine, levetiracetam, oxcarbazepine, pregabalin, tiagabine, topiramate, valproate and zonisamide) used as mono- and adjunctive therapies. Patients who were randomised to receive one of the AEDs had almost twice the risk of suicidal behaviour or ideation (0.43%) compared to patients randomised to receive placebo (0.24%). This risk was generally consistent among the eleven drugs, was observed as early as one week after starting AED and throughout the observed duration of AED treatment and was higher in the clinical trials for epilepsy compared to trials for psychiatric or other conditions.

> *The increased risk of suicidal thoughts or behavior was generally consistent among the eleven drugs with varying mechanisms of action and across a range of indications. This observation suggests that the risk applies to all antiepileptic drugs used for any indication. All patients who are currently taking or starting on any AED for any indication should be monitored for notable changes in behaviour that could indicate the emergence or worsening of suicidal thoughts or behavior or depression.[111]*

However, the problem of suicide and depression in epilepsies, which both have a high incidence, is complicated by a number of factors such as pre-existing psychopathology, social, personal, family and occupational difficulties, teenage onset, and others that have been recently detailed.[112–116] There is no evidence that one AED is more prone than another AED to cause suicidal ideation and suicide.

Common CNS-related ADRs

CNS-related ADRs are common and primarily affect vigilance (somnolence, sedation), cognition, the brain stem and vestibulocerebellar system (leading to dizziness, vertigo, incoordination, ataxia, diplopia or nystagmus), the extrapyramidal system (causing chorea and dystonia, parkinsonism or tremor), or the psychiatric and psychological state of the patient (leading to anxiety, depression, psychosis, and psychological and behavioural disturbances).[117,118] Headache and fatigue are among the commoner CNS-related ADRs of AEDs.

Most of the common CNS ADRs such as sedation, dizziness, incoordination and fatigue are often dose related and occur early after the introduction of an AED. They are reversible, improve with time and can be lessened with slow titration. However, others, such as phenytoin-induced ataxia, appear with long use and are progressive if the responsible agent is not withdrawn. The sedative effect of most older generation AEDs such as phenobarbital and benzodiazepines are well known.

A meta-analysis of the most frequent treatment-emergent CNS ADRs of some new AEDs in adult patients[118] showed significant association of:

- somnolence with gabapentin, levetiracetam, pregabalin , topiramate and zonisamide
- dizziness with gabapentin, lamotrigine, pregabalin, topiramate and zonisamide
- ataxia with lamotrigine and pregabalin
- diplopia with lamotrigine
- fatigue with pregabalin and topiramate
- cognitive impairment with topiramate

Cognitive impairment is common in epilepsies as the result of the seizures, their underlying cause and ADRs to AEDs.[119–123] Cognitive impairment is often of more concern and more debilitating than the actual seizures with a severe impact on quality of life. AEDs may affect any domain of cognition (intelligence, language, visuoperceptual, verbal and nonverbal memory, or executive function) and influence the functional ability of the patient in communication, verbal fluency, problem solving, memory, psychomotor speed and dexterity.

Cognitive ADRs are well known for the older AEDs; it is because of these the use of phenobarbital has been practically prohibited in industrialised countries and particularly the UK. Carbamazepine and valproate are considered to be better than phenytoin in this respect but worse than most of the newer AEDs in RCTs. The relative incidence of cognitive ADRs to newer AEDs are not well known, primarily because of the scarcity of comparative large-scale studies, though topiramate and zonisamide have been associated with significant diffuse cognitive as well as specific ADRs on language and memory. In a recent study attempting to determine the relative prevalence and predictors of subjective cognitive impairment in adult outpatients with epilepsy taking commonly used AEDs (carbamazepine, clobazam, gabapentin, lamotrigine, levetiracetam, oxcarbazepine, phenytoin, topiramate, valproate and zonisamide), overall 320 of 1694 (18.9%) patients experienced cognitive ADRs to AEDs at any point.[119] The average rate of such ADRs for a given AED was 16.6%, with 12.8% leading to dosage change or discontinuation (intolerability). The highest rate of intolerable ADRs was attributed to topiramate (21.5% intolerability) folowed by zonisamide (14.9%), oxcarbazepine (11.6%), levetiracetam (10.4%), carbamazepine (9.9%), lamotrigine (8.9%), valproate (8.3%) and gabapentin (7.3%).

Rates of intolerable ADRs were lower in monotherapy than polytherapy. The highest rate of intolerable cognitive impairment attributed to AEDs in monotherapy was seen with topiramate (11.1%), and was significantly higher than that of carbamazepine (1.5%) or valproate (0.0%).[119]

Significant predictors of ADRs with AEDs are older age, female gender, focal epilepsy, and presence of CNS infection, chronic obstructive pulmonary disease, or other comorbid conditions. Interestingly, the presence/history of static encephalopathy was negatively correlated with such ADRs.[119]

To minimise the risk of drug-induced cognitive dysfunction, "topiramate should be lowest on the list followed by zonisamide and phenytoin, whereas lamotrigine, levetiracetam, gabapentin, valproate and carbamazepine should be higher on the list".[119] Avoidance of phenobarbital is a well known recommendation, which may now be updated to include topiramate and zonisamide.

Behavioural and psychiatric ADRs to AED[124–131]

Patients treated with any AED for any indication should be monitored for the emergence or worsening of depression, suicidal thoughts or behavior, and/or any unusual changes in mood or behavior. (FDA warning for all AEDs)[111]

Evaluating the psychiatric and behavioural ADRs of AEDs is complicated by several factors including the relatively high rate of psychiatric comorbidities in epilepsies, the lack of reliable face to face comparisons and the variety of quality and methods used to assess the occurrence and severity of psychiatric symptoms with AEDs.[124] It is possible that such ADRs are related to the epilepsy itself, to clinical characteristics of more vulnerable patients and some particular properties of the AED itself either alone in monotherapy or in combination with another AED.[125,132]

A current expert opinion is that most psychiatric ADRs primarily occur with rapid titration and high doses for most AEDs.[124] However, such events may happen at any dose, specifically with barbiturates, topiramate, levetiracetam and zonisamide. With the latter AEDs, psychiatric ADRs seem not to occur at random but they are most likely to affect patients with an inherent vulnerability to psychiatric disorders who have a personal or family history of psychiatric illness. In a recent report,[125] the risk of depressive illness associated with topiramate was fivefold higher in patients who underwent rapid titration and this was increased to 23.3-fold in patients with a history of depression.

The paradox is that AEDs are commonly utilised for nonepileptic psychiatric disorders, though there is, in general, a paucity of published RCTs.[133] The overall view is that lamotrigine has antidepressant properties; carbamazepine, valproate, lamotrigine, and oxcarbazepine have mood stabilising properties; and gabapentin, pregabalin, and tiagabine have anxiolytic benefits. Barbiturates, topiramate, and possibly phenytoin may precipitate or exacerbate depression. Underlying depression and anxiety symptoms may be exacerbated by levetiracetam, while psychotic symptoms have rarely been reported with topiramate, levetiracetam, and zonisamide.[133] However, this contradicts firstly with the FDA view that "there is no evidence that one AED is more prone than another AED to cause suicidal ideation and depression"[111] and secondly with the finding that "well-defined DSM-IV disorders are more frequent with topiramate than levetiracetam".[125]

Another paradox is what is known as *forced normalisation* (or alternative psychosis). This is the rare occurrence of psychotic symptoms when the EEG is normalised and seizures have significantly reduced or undergone remission in some patients treated with AEDs for intractable epilepsies.[134] Paranoid psychosis or episodes of major depression are the most frequent manifestations. Forced normalisation has been reported following the use of various AEDs, including phenytoin, carbamazepine, ethosuximide, lamotrigine and levetiracetam.

This is another significant area in which there are more unknowns than knowns and where clinical practice is influenced by reputation rather than concrete evidence.

Non-CNS ADRs of AEDs

ADRs affecting organs outside the CNS are less common and less predictable than those affecting the CNS system but are equally important to recognise because of their impact on physical health and the brain. They affect any body system, including the cardiovascular, integumentary, hematopoetic, hepatic and digestive, renal, metabolic, endocrine, and peripheral nervous systems. They are sometimes difficult to differentiate from other diseases prior to attributing them to a specific AED medication. I have seen many patients investigated invasively and treated for symptoms typical of ADRs to AEDs prior to their recognition as such and their remission after withdrawal of the offensive agent.

Non-CNS ADRs to AEDs may occur soon after the introduction of an AED but they may also happen at a slow and progressive pace during chronic AED treatment. Non-CNS ADRs may also be inconspicuous for many years before they become manifest, sometimes with horrendous consequences.

Adverse cardiac effects of AEDs

There is a conspicuous poverty of information and recommendations on cardiac ADRs of AEDs and their effect on the electrocardiogram (ECG).

The situation may now change in view of the increasing number of studies on SUDEP and the attention now given to cardiac function when assessing drug safety during the regulatory process, particularly with respect to ventricular repolarisation as reflected in the prolongation of the ECG QT interval Premarketing investigation of the safety of a new pharmaceutical agent now includes rigorous characterisation of its effects on the QT/QTc interval labelled "Thorough QT/QTc Study".

The QT interval represents the duration of ventricular depolarisation and subsequent repolarisation, and is measured from the beginning of the QRS complex to the end of the T wave (see Figure 1.2). Prolongation of the QT/QTc interval indicates delay in cardiac repolarisation, which is associated with increased susceptibility to cardiac arrhythmias such as torsade de pointes (torsades) and other ventricular tachyarrhythmias. Torsades is a polymorphic ventricular tachyarrhythmia that can degenerate into ventricular fibrillation, leading to sudden death. Patients with the long QT syndrome may suffer torsades and sudden death. Long QT syndrome is an ion channelopathy that may imitate epileptic seizures; not all carriers of mutated ion channel genes will manifest QT/QTc interval prolongation and polymorphisms can affect ion channels, leading to an increased sensitivity to drugs that affect ventricular repolarisation.

QT prolongation is a rare adverse effect that is seen with many psychotropic drugs including tricyclic antidepressants (with whom carbamazepine is chemically related).[135] There are no AEDs in the long list of drugs implicated in long QT,[136] though carbamazepine and phenytoin have been cited in some reports.[137]

Useful information

Recent regulatory requirements for cardiac safety of drugs

The regulatory concerns regarding cardiac safety of drugs is addressed with the introduction of the International Conference on Harmonisation topic E 14 (ICH-E14) now required by both FDA (http://www.fda.gov/downloads/RegulatoryInformation/Guidances/UCM129357.pdf) and EMEA (http://www.emea.europa.eu/pdfs/human/ich/31013308en.pdf).

The ICH-E14 requires a thorough premarketing investigation of the safety of a new pharmaceutical agent that should include rigorous characterisation of its effects on the QT/QTc interval.

Also, questions have been recently raised regarding the safety and proarrhythmic consequences of drugs that shorten the QT interval.[138] QT shortening has been reported for primidone,[139,140] lamotrigine and rufinamide.[141] As with QT/QTc prolongation, there are genetic syndromes and pharmaceutical agents

Reading an ECG

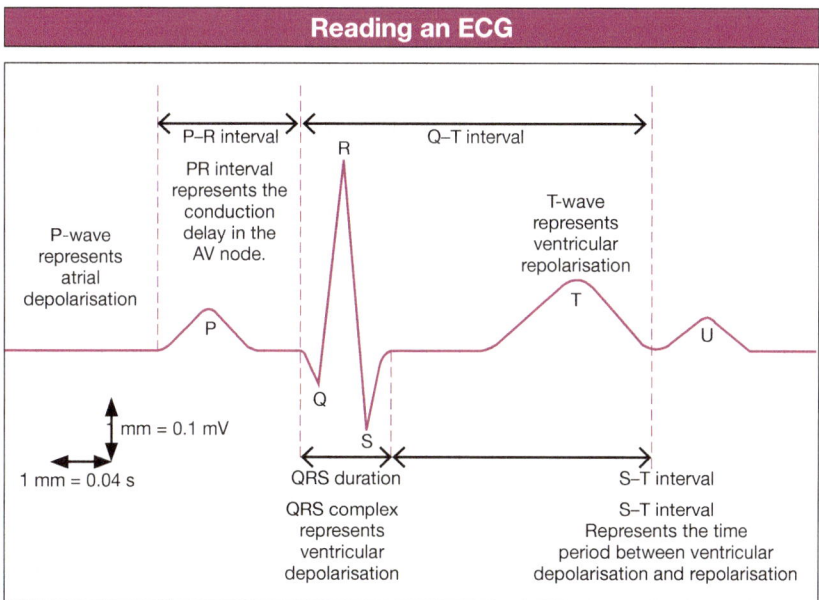

Figure 1.2 The surface ECG represents the different electrophysiological events occurring during normal cardiac conduction. 5 mm = 0.2 s and 0.5 mV.

which cause shortening of QT/QTc. However, currently it is unclear whether QT/QTc shortening is a suitable biomarker for cardiac arrhythmias and how much shortening of QT/QTc is required before it might be considered a safety issue.[138,141]

The PR interval extends from the onset of atrial depolarisation (beginning of the P wave) and ends at the onset of the QRS complex (beginning of ventricular depolarisation) and represents the time the impulse takes to reach the ventricles from the sinus node. The normal values of PR interval are between 0.12 to 0.20 s.

Prolongation of the PR interval of more than 0.20 s (first-degree atrioventricular block) is usually asymptomatic and frequently encountered in clinical practice.[142] Adverse events with first degree atrioventricular block include syncope and bradycardia, which are usually considered of good prognosis. AEDs that are implicated in the prolongation of PR interval are carbamazepine, eslicarbazepine acetate, lacosamide, and pregabalin. Also "a small increase in PR (0.005 seconds)" has been reported in a RCT with lamotrigine.[143]

> *The newest AEDs, including eslicarbazepine acetate, lacosamide and*
> *rufinamide, have been tested after the implementation of ICH-E14, which*
> *may explain why an effect on ECG has been shown in all of these, in contrast*
> *with most other AEDs, which were approved before the ICH-E14 requirements*
> *came into force (Table 1.13).*

Despite their significance in clinical practice, no recommendations on the ECG and cardiac effects of AEDs are made, even in formal guidelines, including those from the National Institute for Health and Clinical Excellence (which only

ECG changes and cardiac adverse reactions of AEDs

AED	Adverse cardiac reactions to AEDs as cited in the SmPCs
Carbamazepine	Cardiac conduction disorders, hypertension or hypotension, bradycardia, arrhythmia, atrioventricular block with syncope, circulatory collapse, congestive heart failure, aggravation of coronary artery disease, thrombophlebitis, thrombo-embolism (e.g. pulmonary embolism)
Eslicarbazepine acetate	PR prolongation
Gabapentin	Palpitations
Lacosamide	PR prolongation
Pregabalin	Tachycardia, atrioventricular block first degree, sinus tachycardia, sinus arrhythmia, sinus bradycardia, congestive heart failure
Rufinamide	Shortening of the QT interval
Lamotrigine, levetiracetam, phenytoin,topiramate, valproate, zonisamide	None is reported in the SmPCs

Table 1.13 Effects of AEDs on ECGs and cardiac ADRs as cited in SmPCs.

states that ECG is recommended when a diagnosis of epilepsy is suspected)[2] and the AES/AAN.[144,145]

Neurologists treating patients with epilepsies have little information on the possible adverse effects of AEDs on cardiac conduction. A common practice is to refer those patients with a known or suspected cardiac or ECG abnormality to a cardiologist when the diagnosis of epilepsy is uncertain or when these 'vulnerable' patients need AED treatment, particularly with carbamazepine.

I find it difficult to draw any firm conclusions from the actual documentation for AEDs (old and new) on ECG changes and cardiac abnormalities; most are anecdotal, hypothetical (based on their mode of action), or based on animal data, case reports or series of case reports. The only relevant review, which just refers to carbamazepine and phenytoin, was published 10 years ago.[146] Even in RCTs, ECG methodology, assessment and results are often unclear. The best one can usually find is the observation that "ECG changes were not of clinical significance". The ECG and cardiac effects of AEDs in neonates and infants are even more difficult to assess. This is reflected even in the carbamazepine publications (the AED in which ECG/cardiac effects are most discussed) as cited by Saetre et al.[147] In one recent report purposely designed to compare effects of lamotrigine with carbamazepine in newly diagnosed elderly patients with epilepsy,[147,148] the main conclusion was that "clinically significant ECG changes are not common during treatment with either of these drugs in elderly patients with no pre-existing significant AV conduction defects" and that the ECG changes were minor and comparable in the two groups. Target maintenance doses were relatively low (400 mg/day for carbamazepine and 100 mg/day for lamotrigine). Nearly 20% of the patients' ECGs were "nonevaluable due to incomplete ECG data" despite the fact that "the highest quality ECG recording equipment had to be used, and that a repeat ECG could be obtained immediately if the quality of the recording was deemed inadequate".[148] No ECG results are reported in the final RCT report of this study.[148]

There is little information on the effect of AEDs in patients with cardiac co-morbidities or those also taking other medications or substances that affect the ECG (including alcohol). Indeed, such patients may be included in RCTs of AEDs and may affect the results one way or the other depending on how many are in the active drug and placebo groups. Another point is that the active drug may have a synergistic effect with other AEDs (such as carbamazepine), which may affect the ECG in add-on RCTs.

Most studies of the ECG/cardiac ADRs of AEDs point out those drugs that inhibit voltage-gated sodium channels, such as phenytoin, carbamazepine and lamotrigine. Also, particular attention has been drawn to drugs (including AEDs)[149] that inhibit the rapid component of the cardiac delayed rectifier potassium ion current (Ikr) expressed by the human hERG gene, because this may increase the risk of cardiac arrhythmia and SUDEP.[150–153] The IKr is also of major importance for embryonic cardiac repolarisation and therefore AEDs that affect the IKr may increase teratogenicity.[154]

Principles of Management in Women with Epilepsies

In medicine, the differences between male and female extend beyond the reproductive hormones and organs. Certain diseases affect women exclusively or predominantly, and there can be significant differences between the sexes in the expression of the same medical problem, and in the response and adverse reactions to drugs.

The way in which epilepsies affect many aspects of a woman's life differs from how they affect men. Women are predisposed towards certain seizure disorders, and antiepileptic drugs (AEDs) can affect physical appearance, the menstrual cycle, contraception, fertility, pregnancy, the unborn baby and the menopause. There is a significant lack of knowledge about and even misunderstanding of many of these issues that are specific to women. These topics have been detailed by expert authors in *Epilepsies in girls and women* (2008), which I co-edited with Pamela Crawford and Torbjörn Tomson,[155] and in "*The XX factor. Treating Women with Antiepileptic Drugs*" by Jim Morrow.[156] This chapter deals only with the clinical implications and demands of AED treatment in women of childbearing age. These issues have also been addressed by a recent practice parameter of the American Academy of Neurology (AAN) and the American Epilepsy Society (AES), which is a three-part evidence-based review focusing on pregnancy in women with epilepsy,[157–159] by an Italian consensus conference on epilepsy and pregnancy, labour and the puerperium,[160] and by other excellent, recently published reviews.[161–178]

The decision to start AED treatment and the choice of AEDs in women with epilepsy requires careful assessment of individual risk in terms of both seizures and adverse (short- or long-term) drug reactions in the patient and her offspring. The main challenge is to offer her an accurate and holistic estimate of the individual risks. Stopping AED medication is equally challenging and often necessary, although it may involve risks of seizure recurrence. The ultimate decision should be taken by a well-informed patient.

Oral hormonal contraception and AEDs[179–181]

Many AEDs interact with oral hormonal contraception with two main consequences:

- contraceptive failure leading to an unplanned pregnancy
- deterioration of seizure control.

C.P. Panayiotopoulos, *Principles of Therapy in the Epilepsies*,
© Springer-Verlag London Limited 2011

Effect of AEDs on oral hormonal contraception

The most commonly used current oral hormonal contraceptives contain 20–35 µg of ethinyloestradiol and less than 1 mg of progestogen. The major part of the oestrogen compound is hydroxylated to inactive metabolites by the hepatic CYP3A4 enzyme or directly conjugated. Hepatic enzyme inducers (see Table 1.6) accelerate hepatic elimination of oral hormonal contraception, which may lead to contraceptive failure. Intramenstrual bleeding is an indicator of contraceptive failure, but does not always occur. There is no substantial risk of contraceptive failure with AEDs other than the hepatic enzyme-inducing drugs.

Women taking hepatic enzyme-inducing AEDs who require contraception should be advised to use:

- high-dose preparations containing at least 50 µg or more of the oestrogen compound
- barrier or other methods of contraception.

Progesterone-only contraception is not an option, because of high failure rates.

During treatment with lamotrigine, the levonorgestrel (synthetic progestogen) component of the oral contraceptive is reduced by about 18%, but this interaction is considered to have no clinical significance; the pharmacokinetics of ethinyloestradiol are unaffected.

Effect of oral hormonal contraception on AEDs

The main AED affected by oral contraception is lamotrigine. Increased glucuronidation of lamotrigine, largely by the progestogen component of oral hormonal contraception, leads to increased elimination of lamotrigine and therefore a decrease in plasma levels of more than 50%. In the pill-free period, plasma lamotrigine levels increase rapidly by 25–50%, which may lead to seizure deterioration and toxicity, but with minor, if any, risk of contraceptive failure. The effect of oral hormonal contraception on other currently used AEDs that undergo glucuronidation is probably of no clinical significance.

Pregnancy

The outlook for pregnant women with epilepsy and their offspring is excellent. The risks to mothers and their babies are small and often preventable. Overall, 95% of women with epilepsy have uncomplicated pregnancies and deliver normal babies. This rate can be significantly improved with proper management; any serious harm to the baby or mother, particularly if it is avoidable, is too much for the family that is affected.

AED treatment during pregnancy is considered necessary for most women with epilepsy, because uncontrolled maternal convulsive seizures pose a greater risk to the fetus than the use of AEDs and may also harm the mother.[161,182] It is also important to remember that the concentration of AEDs may change significantly during pregnancy and the puerperium resulting in an increase in seizures or toxicity.[183,184]

Prescribing AEDs for women with epilepsy may be influenced by marketing and publishing practices that are more likely to favour the newer AEDs.

Recent studies have not indicated any increased risk of obstetric complications in women with epilepsy.

Teratogenicity

It is generally accepted that AED treatment during the first trimester of pregnancy is associated with a small, but significant, increase in the risk of major congenital malformations (MCM) (Tables 2.1 and 2.2). The following statements are as close to reality as I could assess through an extensive review of the literature, which is often unclear. The risk of MCM is:

- probably no different or only slightly higher than the background rate (around 1–2%, see below) in women with epilepsy who are not taking AEDs
- probably less than twice the background rate with commonly used AEDs (other than valproate) as monotherapy, although the relative risk may vary with individual AEDs
- certainly increased with valproate monotherapy to 3–5 times the background rate
- likely to be high with topiramate, though the relevant studies are still inadequate
- certainly higher with polytherapy than monotherapy; valproate is a significant contributor to the high risk of MCM in polytherapy, particularly in combination with lamotrigine (10%)
- likely to be dose dependent, at least for valproate and lamotrigine (i.e. the higher the plasma AED concentration, the higher the relative risk of MCM).

Teratogenicity, teratogenesis and teratogenic (teras = monster) are terms that should be discouraged as inaccurate and derogatory. The expansion of this term to '*cognitive teratogenesis*' as adopted by the AAN/AES[158] is even more inappropriate.

The reported incidence of MCM varies significantly by around 20-fold, mainly because of methodological differences and deficiencies. Earlier studies usually rely on small numbers of recruited patients and lack statistical power. To understand the extent of the difficulties, a total of 722 drug-exposed pregnancies is needed to identify a seven-fold increase in the rate of occurrence of a specific abnormality, such as spina bifida, with a frequency of 1 in 1000[187] or if drug A has a 3% risk for MCM and drug B doubles the risk to 6%, then 750 patients on monotherapy are needed in each group to reach $p < 0.05$ at 80% power. Several large prospective pregnancy registries throughout the world are collecting data on AED-related MCM and other pregnancy-related outcomes in women with epilepsy.[163] However, even these registries have important methodological differences in recruitment, ascertainment, inclusion/exclusion criteria, malformation classification and follow-up that may influence the results and prevent meaningful pooling of data.[177]

Useful clarification on pregnancy C and D categorisation of AEDs

Category D drugs are those drugs for which teratogenicity was seen in both animal and human pregnancies; phenytoin, carbamazepine and valproate are category D drugs. Category C drugs have demonstrated teratogenicity in animals, but the risk in humans is not known. However, this categorisation may be misleading if it is not understood that it is based on changing evidence and that most of the newer AEDs have not been assessed. For example, carbamazepine is a class D drug though the risk of MCM may be equal or less than that with lamotrigine or topiramate.

It may be too early to draw definite conclusions for the new-generation AEDs, all of which are classified as category C, with the exception of lamotrigine, which is downgraded to category D in Australia.[185] Also, with the exception of topiramate and vigabatrin, the newer AEDs do not appear to be teratogenic in animals when administered in subtoxic doses.[186]

Background rate of MCM is generally considered to be 1–2%, but reports vary. The Active Malformation Surveillance Program at Brigham and Women's Hospital in Boston, USA, estimates the background rate to be 1.6% after exclusion of genetic and chromosomal anomalies.[188] Some use the higher rate of 3.2%[189] determined by the Metropolitan Atlanta Congenital Defects Program,[190] but this population-based registry uses active case identification from multiple sources, undertakes direct chart review of potential cases and includes all malformations identified up to the age of 5 years.[191]

Commonly used older generation AEDs and major congenital malformations

Valproate is definitely associated with an elevated risk for MCM (Tables 2.1 and 2.2), including a 10-fold increase in spina bifida aperta (1–2% of infants exposed). The risk is dose-related, particularly at doses of more than 1000 mg/day. Polytherapy with valproate and any other AED is highly teratogenic and appears to be even worse in combination with lamotrigine (1 of 10 infants exposed).[189,192]

MCM rates after exposure to commonly used older AEDs[178]

AED	Range (%)	Mean ± SD (%)
Carbamazepine	1.4–11.4	4.9 ± 1.5
Phenobarbital	2.8–16.7	7.0 ± 4.2
Phenytoin	0.0–16.0	5.0 ± 3.0
Valproate	5.7–17.4	10.9 ± 3.9

Table 2.1

Major congenital malformation in pregnancy registers

	Number of women with epilepsy		MCM (%)		95% CI	
	UK Epilepsy Pregnancy Register[†]	North American Epilepsy Pregnancy Register[‡]	UK Epilepsy Pregnancy Register	North American Epilepsy Pregnancy Register	UK Epilepsy Pregnancy Register	North American Epilepsy Pregnancy Register
No exposure to AEDs	445		2.2		1.2–4.1	
Exposure to AEDs	5475		3.9		3.4–7.2	
Monotherapy	4276		3.4		2.9–4.9	
Monotherapy with valproate	1097		5.8		4.5–7.4	
Monotherapy with carbamazepine	1444	873	2.4	2.6	1.7–3.3	1.5–4.3
Monotherapy with lamotrigine	1524	684	2.4	2.3	1.7–3.3	1.3–3.8
Monotherapy with levetiracetam	177	197	0	2	0.0–2.3	0.65–4.8
Monotherapy with topiramate	92	197	4.8	4.1	1.9–7.6	1.9–7.6
Polytherapy (> 130 AED combinations)	1199		5.8		4.6–7.2	
Polytherapy with valproate*	451		8.6		6.4–11.6	
Polytherapy with carbamazepine	526		4.9		3.4–7.1	
Polytherapy with lamotrigine	644		5.3		3.8–7.3	
Polytherapy with levetiracetam	229		3.9		2.1–7.3	
Polytherapy with topiramate	162		8.6		5.2–14.0	

Table 2.2 *Polytherapy with valproate had a significantly higher rate of MCM (8.6%) than regimens without valproate (odds ratio 2.3; 95% CI 1.4–3.7). [†]Data courtesy of Dr. Jim Morrow and the UK Epilepsy and Pregnancy Register. [‡]Data provided at http://www2.massgeneral.org/aed/newsletter/Winter2009newsletter.pdf.

Considering that valproate is possibly also associated with cognitive impairment of infants exposed to this drug during pregnancy,[193] it should be avoided in women with epilepsy of childbearing age. This is not a setback for women with focal epilepsies as there are many other AEDs that are more effective and less teratogenic than valproate; valproate should never have been promoted as equivalent to carbamazepine for the treatment of women with focal seizures.[282] The real problem is for women with generalised epilepsies such as JME in whom very few other AEDs are effective; alternatives are probably restricted to levetiracetam (most likely to be effective and less likely to be teratogenic) and lamotrigine (most popular but associated with significant problems to be considered in women with epilepsy and worsening of myoclonic seizures). Some authorities also consider that small doses of valproate may be recommended in some women of childbearing age with uncontrolled primarily GTCS and JME.

Avoid entirely valproate polytherapy in any combination and particularly with lamotrigine. The risks are high and outweigh any benefits.

Carbamazepine is classified as a pregnancy category D drug, but recent evidence indicates that the rate of MCM is not a significant concern in relation to other AEDs (Tables 2.1 and 2.2).[158] Therefore, the previously emphasised[194] association of carbamazepine with a significant increase in spina bifida aperta (0.5%)has to be reassessed. Carbamazepine probably does not increase poor cognitive outcomes compared to unexposed controls.[158]

Phenobarbital and phenytoin are considered to have definite, but relatively low, teratogenicity in relation to valproate (Tables 2.1 and 2.2).[158] However, both drugs have also been implicated as possibly causing cognitive impairment in exposed infants,[158] though this was based on a few class II and III studies and has not been replicated in a more recent study (see cognitive teratogenesis below).[193] Nevertheless, phenytoin should be avoided in women with epilepsy, because of aesthetic and other ADRs.[194]

Clonazepam and clobazam. There is no evidence of a significant increase in teratogenicity in women with epilepsy receiving monotherapy with clonazepam or clobazam.[195–198]

Commonly used new generation of broad spectrum AEDs and major congenital malformations

The risks for MCM with most new generation AEDs have not been assessed. Based on existing evidence, the risks associated with three of the more widely used broad spectrum AEDs – lamotrigine, levetiracetam and topiramate (Table 2.2) – are as follows.

Lamotrigine. Significant differences in the risk for MCM have been reported by two of the largest pregnancy registries, though the rate of MCM was similar (2.3–2.4%).[187,192,199] The UK Epilepsy and Pregnancy Register noted a positive dose-response relationship for MCMs with lamotrigine (p = 0.006) with a MCM rate of 5.4% (95% CI 3.3–8.7%) for total daily doses of more than 200 mg. This

MCM rate was similar to that in those receiving valproate at a dose of 1000 mg or less (5.1%; 95% CI 3.5–7.3). While there was a trend towards lamotrigine being associated with fewer MCMs than valproate, the differences were minimised in those infants exposed to a dose of lamotrigine of more than 200 mg each day.[192] The North American AED pregnancy registry reported a 10.4-fold increase (95% CI 4.3–24.9) in isolated cleft palate or cleft lip deformity,[187] but this has not been confirmed in the UK[199] and the European Surveillance of Congenital Anomalies (EUROCAT) registers.[200]

The international lamotrigine pregnancy registry concluded that "the risk of all major birth defects after first trimester exposure to lamotrigine monotherapy (2.9%) was similar to that in the general population",[189] but this was considered to be an overestimate by other authorities, who suggested that a more accurate conclusion may be "the risk for major malformations associated with first trimester exposure to lamotrigine is only about twice that of the general population... when similar definitions, inclusions and case identification strategies are used".[191] Furthermore, it would be even more difficult to assess the risks of MCM with lamotrigine precisely without TDM, if the finding of a dose-related effect[192] is replicated, because of the significant decrease in plasma levels of lamotrigine (nearly by 50%) in the first trimester of pregnancy.

In polytherapy with lamotrigine and other AEDs, the risk of MCM is 5.3% (95% CI 3.8–7.3) (Table 2.2) and this doubles to around 10% in combination with valproate.[189,192]

Alarmingly, lamotrigine and valproate is the most frequently used AED combination in pregnancy according to the recent EURAP report,[201] despite the fact that it may harm 1 in 10 exposed babies. This is twice the frequency seen with any other combination and indicates a lack of information reaching those prescribing AEDs for women; the messages either do not get through or are unclear.

Lamotrigine has been downgraded to pregnancy category D by the Australian regulatory administration.[185]

Levetiracetam. The number of women treated with levetiracetam in pregnancy registries is still too small to draw definite conclusions, but the data from the UK Epilepsy and Pregnancy Register are very encouraging (Table 2.2).[202] Not a single MCM has been seen in the offspring of 133 women receiving levetiracetam monotherapy (95% CI 0.0–2.8) and the risk of MCM was relatively small (3.9%) in 229 women receiving polytherapy with levetiracetam and other AEDs (95% CI 2.1–7.3).

Topiramate. The use of topiramate in women of childbearing age is uncertain but in my assessment it should probably not be given to this group of patients unless absolutely necessary. This is because topiramate is (a) teratogenic in animals even at subtoxic doses (equivalent to 0.2–10 times the therapeutic doses recommended in humans)[186,203] and (b) has serious ADRs that are likely to affect the fetus, because of the extensive transplacental transfer of the drug. Preliminary results may indicate that such precautions are justified.[203,204] In the UK Epilepsy and Pregnancy Register (Table 2.2), the MCM rate in 79 women receiving topiramate monotherapy was 3.8% (95% CI 1.3–10.6) and in 162 women receiving polytherapy was 8.6% (95% CI 5.2–14). The rate of MCM was even higher (9.8%) in one report of 41 live births from 52 pregnancies during topiramate treatment (29 on monotherapy and and 23 on polytherapy);[203] this finding has, however, been undermined by statistical deficiencies.[205] However, animal studies are not certain predictors of human teratogenicity and the numbers of women studied are still small and need to be statistically verified in pregnancy registries. At the risk of being overcautious, it may be too dangerous to wait for the outcome in thousands of women receiving topiramate in order to validate the teratogenic potential of this drug.

Oxcarbazepine. There is practically no evidence of the teratogenic potential with oxcarbazepine, though preliminary results indicate that this may not be significant.[176] However, oxcarbazepine is associated with an increase in seizure frequency during pregnancy, probably because of the significant 26–38% decrease in levels of its active monohydroxy derivative.[206]

Clarifications and limitations of the AAN/AES report

The AAN/AES review is a laudable endeavour by leaders in the field to provide us with an evidence-based assessment of this important and difficult topic. However, such reports have significant limitations in clinical practice as detailed in "evidence based recommendations" (pages 25–30). In this occasion, the AAN/AES report has the following drawbacks:

(a) It is already outdated, because the assessed evidence was published from December 2005 through to February 2008. More recent evidence-based reports cited in this book have not been included, although some of them that contradict or reinforce the AAN/AES conclusions would probably require an Addendum. An example of this is detailed in the next page of the section "Post-natal cognitive effects of foetal exposure to AEDs."

(b) Evidence of "an increased risk of isolated oral clefts in infants born to mothers exposed to lamotrigine monotherapy in the first trimester of pregnancy" was not considered, despite the warnings from the manufacturer issued in April 2006, which prompted its degrading to category pregnancy D by the Australian authorities.[185] Nor did the report consider other data on levetiracetam and topiramate reviewed in this book.

The AAN/AES assessments of AED-related MCMs

The recent AAN/AES assessments made the following key conclusions.[158]

- AEDs taken during the first trimester probably increase the risk of MCMs in the offspring of women with epilepsy, but it cannot be determined if the increased risk is imparted by all AEDs, or only one or some AEDs.
- Valproate monotherapy during the first trimester possibly increases the risk of MCMs in the offspring of women with epilepsy.

- Valproate used in polytherapy probably increases the risk of MCMs in the offspring of women with epilepsy.
- Carbamazepine probably does not substantially increase the risk of MCMs in the offspring of women with epilepsy.
- There is insufficient evidence to determine whether lamotrigine or other specific AEDs increase the risk of MCMs in the offspring of women with epilepsy.

Foetal anticonvulsant syndrome and minor anomalies

Many reports associate intrauterine exposure to a specific AED with a cluster of foetal abnormalities constituting a specific foetal anticonvulsant syndrome (e.g. phenytoin, carbamazepine, valproate foetal anticonvulsant syndrome).[207] The foetal anticonvulsant syndrome manifests with various abnormalities including intrauterine growth retardation, MCM, cognitive and behavioural impairment, and a number of minor anomalies such as craniofacial dysmorphisms (hypertelorism, flat nasal ridge, low-set ears, microcephaly, short neck) and digital anomalies (hypoplasia of the distal phalanges or nails). Though some of these features are more prominent in association with one AED compared with another, it is now generally accepted that the separation of the various syndromes of embryo-foetal exposure to AEDs is not as clear-cut as previously thought; genetic factors contribute more than individual AEDs to the foetal anticonvulsant syndrome. Minor anomalies are difficult to evaluate prospectively and may occur in isolation from other features.

The finding that some MCMs occur more frequently following exposure to a specific AED also needs to be viewed in context. MCMs seen more frequently with valproate, such as neural tube defects, can also occur following exposure to other AEDs, demonstrating that this is not an AED-specific MCM.

Like other teratogens, AEDs produce a pattern of MCMs with overlap among the individual AEDs.[158]

Post-natal cognitive effects of foetal exposure to AEDs

There is significant uncertainty about the effect of epilepsy and AED therapy on cognition in children born to mothers with epilepsy.[178] In the conclusions of the AAN/AES practice parameter,[158] first, I am discouraged by the term 'cognitive teratogenesis', which is derogatory and inaccurate, and secondly, I, like others,[178] caution that their recommendations may not precisely represent the true dimension of this problem and its route. By the nature of an evidence-based assessment, the AAN/AES conclusions come mainly from class II and III studies, the confounding factors have not been analysed, the recommendations are probable or possible, and older AEDs have mainly been examined although more should now be known about the newer AEDs with increasing numbers of mothers participating in the pregnancy registries. The influence of AEDs with a high rate of adverse cognitive impairment (e.g. topiramate)[119] may be of particular concern.

In the AAN/AES practice parameter,[158] the outcome measure was an assessment of the child's intelligence quotient (IQ) at age 2 years or older. Because maternal IQ is an important influence on child IQ, studies were downgraded if they did not control for maternal IQ. It was also assumed that the cognitive risk was related to AED exposure throughout pregnancy and was not confined to the first trimester. The main conclusions of this AAN/AES report are:

1. Cognition is probably not reduced in children of women with epilepsy who are not exposed to AEDs in utero.
2. There is insufficient evidence to determine whether the children of women with epilepsy taking AEDs in general are at increased risk for reduced cognition.
    *   Cognitive outcomes are probably reduced in children exposed to AED polytherapy compared with monotherapy in utero.
    *   Carbamazepine probably does not increase poor cognitive outcomes compared with unexposed controls.
    *   Valproate is probably associated with poor cognitive outcomes compared with unexposed controls.
    *   Phenytoin is possibly associated with poor cognitive outcomes compared with unexposed controls (the results are, however, conflicting; see below[193]).
    *   Phenobarbital is possibly associated with poor cognitive outcomes in the male offspring of women with epilepsy compared with unexposed controls (the results are, however, conflicting; see below[193]).
    *   Cognitive outcomes are probably reduced in children exposed to valproate during pregnancy compared with carbamazepine and possibly phenytoin.

It is difficult to assess how severely cognition is impaired in these children, but the differences, though significant, may not be extreme. A recent interim report of a prospective, observational, multicentre study in the USA and UK detailed the cognitive outcomes in 309 children at 3 years of age.[193] Contrary to the conclusions of the AES/AAN practice parameters, there were no significant differences between children exposed to phenytoin (IQ 98), carbamazepine (IQ 99) or lamotrigine (IQ 101). However, valproate was associated with a significantly lower IQ (92). The association between valproate use and IQ was dose dependent. Children's IQs were significantly related to maternal IQs among children exposed to carbamazepine, lamotrigine or phenytoin, but not among those exposed to valproate.

Children with intrauterine exposure to high doses of valproate may suffer cognitive impairment, but it would be speculative to state anything further until prospective studies including the newer AEDs are carried out. Such studies also need to consider a significant number of confounding factors, including the occurrence of convulsive seizures that appear to cause cognitive impairment of the infant.

Change in seizure frequency and status epilepticus during pregnancy

In most women with epilepsy, seizure frequency in pregnancy is similar to that before pregnancy. Existing findings do not suggest a great increase in the frequency of seizures or status epilepticus during pregnancy or an increased risk of seizure relapse during pregnancy for women who are seizure-free.[159] This is another compelling reason to strive for improvement and possibly seizure freedom in women with epilepsy who are planning pregnancy.[159]

Significant progress has been made in our understanding of the factors that may predict seizure deterioration or improvement, and recurrence or remission, though they have not been fully elucidated. In most patients (69%), epilepsy largely follows the same pattern as before pregnancy (Table 2.3).[159] Furthermore, most women (84%) who are seizure-free for at least 9 months before pregnancy do not experience any recurrences (Table 2.3). In the minority of women whose epilepsy changes during pregnancy, what happens in the various types of seizures (particularly GTCS, which are the most severe and may harm the unborn baby) and syndromes is largely unknown. Seizure frequency and severity may even vary between different pregnancies in the same patient. I have seen extreme cases of tremendous deterioration or improvement during pregnancy, as well as some exceptional cases in which GTCS occurred only during pregnancy.

Some studies indicate that changes are more likely to occur during the first and the third trimesters, and that seizure frequency tends to revert to pre-pregnancy levels after delivery. Using the first trimester as a reference, seizure control remains unchanged throughout pregnancy in 64% of women, 93% of whom are seizure-free during the entire pregnancy. For those with a change in seizure frequency, 17% have an increase and 16% a decrease in seizure frequency.[208] According to unconfirmed reports, seizure deterioration is higher in focal epilepsies than in generalised epilepsies.[209]

Status epilepticus. There is insufficient evidence to support or refute an increased risk of status epilepticus in pregnancy.[159] However, its prevalence is probably very low, ranging from 0–0.6%, which approximates to an annual prevalence of

Change in seizures during pregnancy. Analysis of data from five studies (n=537) described by the AAN/AES[159]		
	Range (%)	**Mean±SD**
Seizures unchanged	54–80	69 ± 12
Seizures decreased	0.3–24	12 ± 7
Seizures increased	14–32	19 ± 7
Seizure-free rate in 948 women previously seizure-free for > 9 months	74–92	84 ± 8

Table 2.3

0.5-1.6% for convulsive and non-convulsive status epilepticus in patients with various types of epilepsy.[210,211]

Seizure deterioration in pregnancy due to changes in plasma AED concentrations

Seizure deterioration in pregnancy can often be attributed to poor compliance, an inappropriate reduction in AED therapy either by the patient or her physician, a pregnancy-related fall in plasma drug concentrations, sleep deprivation, fatigue, hormonal changes or psychological factors. Patients often decide themselves to reduce or stop AED medication as a result of media concerns.

An important factor in seizure deterioration is inadequate plasma levels of AEDs either because of non-compliance (often compounded by vomiting) or, primarily, because of the multiple physiological changes occurring during pregnancy that influence drug disposition, including increased volume of distribution, increased renal elimination, altered hepatic enzyme activity, and a decline in plasma protein concentrations.[170,183] A decrease in plasma albumin and protein binding, and the displacement of AEDs by endogenous compounds, lead to an alteration in the ratio of total to free drug, which is particularly important for highly protein-bound drugs.[183]

For many AEDs, significant increases in clearance and therefore decreases in plasma levels are charac-teristic during pregnancy.[157,170,209] There is documented evidence of significant increases in the clearance of lamotrigine and phenytoin during pregnancy. The clearance of phenobarbital, the active monohydroxy derivative of oxcarbazepine and levetiracetam also increases during pregnancy.[157,170,183,206]

Women taking lamotrigine have been best studied in this regard. The pronounced decline in plasma concentrations of lamotrigine during pregnancy has been shown to be associated with a deterioration in seizure frequency in more than 50% of patients, such that patients often require dose adjustments[172,212] or additional AEDs.[208] In the Australian pregnancy registry, the control of convulsive seizures was significantly worse with lamotrigine than with valproate (during the entire pregnancy) or carbamazepine (during the second and the third trimester).[212] Oxcarbazepine is the only other AED associated with poorer seizure control.[206,208] Focal epilepsy, polytherapy and oxcarbazepine monotherapy were independently associated with an increase in seizure frequency in the second and third trimester compared with the first trimester.[208] In the most recent report, 8 of 11 women experienced seizure deterioration during the pregnancy, five of whom had previously been seizure free. In seven women (about 50%), seizure frequency at least doubled during pregnancy, and there was a trend towards a correlation between seizure deterioration and the decrease in the plasma concentration of the monohydroxy derivative (MHD).[206]

The AAN/AES[157] has assessed the changes that occur during pregnancy for each AED, as follows:

Lamotrigine. Pregnancy probably increases the clearance and decreases plasma levels of lamotrigine during pregnancy. The decrease in plasma level is associated with an increase in seizure frequency (one class I and two class II studies).

Carbamazepine. Pregnancy probably causes a small decrease in plasma levels of carbamazepine: 9% in the second trimester and 12% in the third trimester (one class I study).

Phenytoin. Pregnancy probably causes an increase in the clearance and a decrease in plasma levels of phenytoin during pregnancy (one class I study).

Oxcarbazepine. Pregnancy possibly causes a decrease in the level of the active monohydroxy derivative of oxcarbazepine (two class III studies).

Levetiracetam. Pregnancy possibly causes a decrease in plasma levels of levetiracetam (one Class II study).

Phenobarbital, valproate, primidone and ethosuximide. Evidence of a change in clearance or plasma levels of phenobarbital, valproate, primidone or ethosuximide during pregnancy is insufficient to reach a conclusion.

Therapeutic drug monitoring *in pregnancy has* been formally recommended as invaluable in pregnant women with epilepsy because of the significant AEDs changes during pregnancy and the puerperium.[78,157,184,213]

This is particularly recommended for:
- lamotrigine, carbamazepine and phenytoin (level B evidence)[157]
- levetiracetam and oxcarbazepine (as monohydroxy derivative) (level C evidence)[157]
- highly protein-bound drugs; free drug concentrations should be measured for phenobarbital, phenytoin, carbamazepine, valproate and primidone.[157, 184,213]

Current published guidelines recommend that the ideal AED concentration should be established for each patient before conception and that monitoring of AED concentrations should be performed during each trimester and in the last month of pregnancy.[78] Some authors recommend at least monthly monitoring of AED concentrations, especially for lamotrigine.[172]

Clinical context of TDM: There is significant evidence to support active monitoring of AED levels during pregnancy. This is especially true for lamotrigine and oxcarbazepine, as changes in levels were associated with an increase in seizure frequency.[206,212] In pueprerium, there is an increase risk of toxicity if levels of certain AEDs had been adjusted during pregnancy but not after delivery. Unfortunately, there are no clear data on the timing of the return to the pre-pregnancy pharmacokinetic state post-partum. One study[214] demonstrated that an empiric post-partum taper schedule of lamotrigine reduced the occurrence of post-partum toxicity, but more systematic information is needed for all AEDs regarding their pharmacokinetic alterations in order to determine the management of AED dosing in the post-partum period.[157]

TDM should be individualised for each patient with the aim of maintaining a level at which seizure control was good. It is expected that such TDM in pregnancy and purperium will improve seizure control but this is not tested.[157]

Excesses or undue reliance on TDM outside their clinical context is discouraged. (See the section on TDM in chapter 1.)

Effect of seizures on mother and the unborn baby

GTCS may cause severe harm to both mother and her unborn baby, but may be preventable with appropriate management.

The harmful effects of seizures, and particularly GTCS, are multiple, and may be severe or even fatal, and may be accidental (falls, drowning) or non-accidental (aspiration, pulmonary oedema, cardiac arrhythmias, cardiac asystole). Furthermore, the risk of sudden unexplained death in epilepsy (SUDEP) is significantly higher in patients with GTCS than in patients with other types of seizure. Pregnancy is a particularly vulnerable period, both for the woman and her unborn baby. In pregnancy, a GTCS imposes an increased risk of damage or death to the mother and her unborn baby. Other types of seizure that may be harmful are those associated with autonomic disturbances and cardiac asystole. The consequences of convulsive status epilepticus are much worse than those of brief seizures. A study in the UK found that the odds for maternal death were approximately 10 times higher for women with epilepsy than for the general population.[215] Case histories have suggested that these extra deaths were due to GTCS that occurred mainly after stopping AEDs or poor compliance (but this is not certain as the case histories were often incomplete).[215]

The harmful effects of seizures on the unborn baby also arise from accidental injury, or the hypoxic and other effects of the seizure on the mother or directly on the fetus (e.g. lactic acidosis, bradycardia). Foetal fatalities may rarely occur during status epilepticus; only one foetus died in 12 pregnancies of women with convulsive status epilepticus, but fortunately with no maternal mortality.[208] The number of stillbirths is not increased among women who are adequately treated for epilepsy during pregnancy.

Seizures during pregnancy are not linked to an increased risk for anatomical malformations in the infant, though one report found a 12.3% malformation rate in women experiencing seizures during the first trimester compared with 4% in women who did not (details and other citations in reference 216). However, maternal GTCS during pregnancy are associated with cognitive deficits,[182] which is another important reason for providing adequate AED treatment.

Labour and delivery. The risk of seizures is particularly high during labour and delivery, and the risk is higher in those who had seizures earlier in pregnancy;[209] 1–2% of women will have a GTCS during labour and a further 1–2% will have a GTCS within the next 24 hours. Women at risk of seizures should be managed in specialised obstetric units with facilities for maternal and neonatal resuscitation.

Obstetric and other pregnancy-related complications

Obstetric and other pregnancy-related complications in women with epilepsy are few and probably not significantly different from those in a control population.[159]

For women taking AEDs, there is probably no substantially increased risk (>2 times expected) of caesarean delivery or late pregnancy bleeding, and probably no moderately increased risk (>1.5 times expected) of premature contractions or premature labour and delivery. There is possibly a substantially increased risk of premature contractions and premature labour and delivery during pregnancy for women who smoke. There is insufficient evidence to support or refute an increase in the risk for pre-eclampsia, pregnancy-related hypertension or spontaneous abortion.[159]

Adverse perinatal outcomes

According to the AAN/AES evidence-based review,[159] neonates of women taking AEDs:

- probably have an increased risk of being small for gestational age (defined as birth weight below the tenth percentile for the study population when adjusted for gestational age and gender) of about twice the expected rate
- possibly have an increased risk of 1-minute Apgar scores below of about twice the expected rate.

There is probably no substantially increased risk of perinatal death in neonates born to women with epilepsy. For other perinatal outcomes, such as respiratory distress, intrauterine growth retardation and admission to a neonatal intensive care unit, data were inadequate to draw conclusions.

The infants of women taking enzyme-inducing AEDs are at potential but probably small risk for haemorrhagic disease.[159] It has therefore been recommended that the mother takes oral phytomenadione (vitamin K1) 10–20 mg/day for at least 1 month before delivery and/or that the infant receives vitamin K1 0.5–1 mg intramuscularly at birth. However, there is no consensus amongst guidelines and recommendations on these matters and the risks involved.

Folic acid supplementation for the prevention of major congenital malformations

Low folate levels are associated with an increased risk of spontaneous abortion and MCMs, including neural tube defects, which is why official health guidelines recommend folic acid supplementation for all women in the general population who might become pregnant. This may prevent neural tube defects in the 72% of women at high risk of giving birth to children with such abnormalities. Whether folic acid supplementation would also reduce AED-related MCM in children of women who are taking AEDs, some of which may have folic acid-antagonist properties, is debatable.[157,217] The AAN/AES assessed that the risk of AED-related MCMs in the offspring of women with epilepsy is possibly reduced by folic acid supplementation and recommended that, although there are still insufficient data, "there is no evidence of harm and no reason to suspect that it would not be effective in this group".[157]

The current recommendation is that all women of childbearing potential, with or without epilepsy, should take a folic acid supplement of at least 0.4 mg/ day (higher doses have also been recommended) before conception (usually starting from when they stop contraception) and during at least the first trimester of pregnancy (until the end of the 12th week of pregnancy).

Foods with high folic acid content include green leafy vegetables (e.g. spinach and spring greens), broccoli, fortified breakfast cereals and brown rice.

For women on AEDs, some authorities recommend bigger doses of folic acid. However, a recent class 1 study of the UK Epilepsy and Pregnancy register found no statistical differences in either MCM or neural tube defects between women with epilepsy who received folic acid before conception and those who did not.[217] The authors concluded that the increased risk of MCM in women taking AEDs probably occurs through mechanisms other than folic acid metabolism.[217]

Breastfeeding and AEDs

Breastfeeding is the ideal way of providing young infants with the nutrients they need for healthy growth and development. Virtually all mothers can breastfeed, provided they have accurate information, and the support of their family and the healthcare system. Colostrum, the yellowish, sticky breast milk produced at the end of pregnancy, is recommended as the perfect food for the newborn, and feeding should be initiated within the first hour after birth. Exclusive breastfeeding is recommended up to 6 months of age.

World Health Organization (WHO)

These WHO recommendations also apply to women with epilepsy who are not taking AEDs. However, for women taking AEDs, the usual advice is that "the benefits of breastfeeding must be weighed against the potential risks of exposing the infant to medications". So how can this balance between benefit and risk be assessed, and how can a physician be certain about the advice to give the mother with so many unknowns? There is no way to determine whether indirect exposure to maternally ingested AEDs has symptomatic effects on the newborn, as there are no controlled studies comparing the newborns of women taking AEDs with those of women not taking AEDs. A drug that is safe for use during pregnancy may not be safe for the nursing infant.[157]

Most AEDs pass into breast milk and some do so in significant quantities (Table 2.4). Medications that are highly protein bound, that have large molecular weights or that are poorly lipid-soluble do not tend to enter the breast milk in clinically important quantities. However, it is clinically important to appreciate that, in the early post-partum period, large gaps between the mammary alveolar cells allow many medications to pass through this milk that may not be able to enter mature milk; these gaps close by the second week of lactation.

The nursing infant's drug exposure depends on the concentration of the drug in the breast milk and the amount of breast milk consumed by the infant. The pharmacological activity of the medication depends on its absorption, distribution, metabolism and elimination, which may differ in the newborn from that in children and adults, and can also vary with different drugs.[218] It is for these reasons that the amount of AED in the breast milk is not always proportional to the *infant/maternal plasma concentration* (Table 2.4). For example, though the concentration of phenobarbital in the maternal milk is 30–50% of that in the maternal plasma, plasma levels in the infant are high (Table 2.4); the converse is true for levetiracetam. A single dose of phenobarbital may persist for days in an infant, because of the slow rate of barbiturate metabolism in this age group, and may cause lethargy, sleepiness or irritability and agitation. On the other hand, an infant who is not breast fed, but whose mother was taking phenobarbital during pregnancy, may experience withdrawal symptoms. Furthermore, repeated administration of a drug such as lamotrigine via breast milk may lead to accumulation in the infant.[219] Probably any drug whose concentration in breast milk is close to 100% that in the maternal plasma can be problematic; however, further data are needed to confirm this.

There is no threshold level of passive exposure to AEDs that has been established to impart a clinically important risk to the fetus or neonate. The panel

AED placental transfer, and amounts in the maternal milk and the infant

AED	
Placental transfer[157]	
Probably potentially clinically important amounts	Carbamazepine, levetiracetam, phenobarbital, phenytoin, primidone, and valproate
Possibly potentially clinically important amounts	Gabapentin, lamotrigine, oxcarbazepine and topiramate
Amounts in maternal milk in relation to plasma levels[218]	
Levels higher or approaching maternal plasma level	Ethosuximide, gabapentin, levetiracetam, topiramate, and zonisamide
Levels 50–80% of maternal plasma level	Lamotrigine, primidone and oxcarbazepine
Levels < 50% of maternal plasma level	Carbamazepine, phenobarbital, phenytoin and valproate
Plasma levels in breastfed infant[218]	
< 20% of maternal levels	Carbamazepine, gabapentin, levetiracetam, oxcarbazepine, phenytoin, topiramate and valproate
> 50% of maternal levels	Ethosuximide and phenobarbital
20–50% of maternal levels	Lamotrigine

Table 2.4

of the AAN/AES stipulated that an AED transfer rate of 0.6 (neonatal:maternal plasma concentration ratio or a milk:maternal concentration ratio) was potentially clinically important, together with any trend of increasing plasma concentrations in the neonate by 25% over the evaluation period (generally 3 days up to 1 month).[157]

Table 2.5 lists AEDs according to whether or not they are considered appropriate for breastfeeding by the WHO and the American Academy of Paediatrics. However, even these recommendations may be debated. For example, many authorities warn of the potential for fatal hepatotoxicity with valproate in children under 2 years of age.

Breastfeeding may be particularly problematic in

- premature or otherwise compromised infants that may require altered dosing to avoid drug accumulation and toxicity[220]
- infants of women receiving AED polytherapy.

Useful note

- The infant's AED exposure can be limited by avoiding breastfeeding during periods of peak maternal plasma drug concentration.
- A breastfeeding mother should never stop her medication abruptly, as she may have seizures and the baby may experience drug withdrawal.
- Signs of AED withdrawal in the baby include increased irritability, insomnia, sweating and seizures.

Principles of AED therapy in women of childbearing age in clinical practice

Finding the balance between optimal therapy to control seizures and the avoidance of adverse effects or other harm to the woman and her offspring is the crux of proper management. Women should be made fully aware of all aspects of AED treatment and be able to make informed decisions. Ultimately, the patient is the decision-maker and the physician the provider of information.

Recommendations on AEDs for breastfeeding women*

Recommendation	AED
Yes	Carbamazepine, ethosuximide, phenytoin and valproate
Yes with caution	Clobazam, clonazepam, gabapentin, lamotrigine, levetiracetam, oxcarbazepine, topiramate and vigabatrin
No	Felbamate
No consensus	Phenobarbital

Table 2.5 *Based on information from Johannessen and Tomson (2008).[218]

The basic principles of AED treatment in all patients also apply to women, but priority should be given to AEDs that are most likely to control seizures and less likely to adversely interfere with the particular needs of women of childbearing age. Efforts should be made to avoid AEDs that may be harmful to women and their offspring. All aspects of the management of epilepsy and the implications for contraception and pregnancy should be thoroughly discussed with the patient, who should also preferably be provided with written information.

Commencing AED therapy in women of childbearing age with newly diagnosed focal epilepsy

Information regarding teratogenic potential is given in Tables 2.1 and 2.2. It may be easier to first exclude AEDs that score worse than others. These are:

Valproate is first in the list of unwanted AEDs in women with focal epilepsies for two reasons. Firstly, it poses significant risks in pregnancy, leads to weight gain and has hormonal effects. Secondly, valproate is not as effective as other AEDs in focal seizures of any type. European epileptologists, including myself, were using valproate effectively as the superior AED for generalised epilepsies; we were not recommending it as a first line option in focal epilepsies, for which carbamazepine was preferred. Unfortunately, this clinical practice was spoiled by subsequent 'evidence-based' reports and meta-analyses that found valproate to be "as effective as carbamazepine" particularly in the UK. This resulted in the widespread use of valproate with detrimental effects at least in those women with focal epilepsy that were treated with the drug.

Phenytoin has numerous ADRs and mainly aesthetic changes, such as gingival hyperplasia, hirsutism and dysmorphia. It is an enzyme inducer and it has been implicated in the so-called 'foetal phenytoin syndrome' (though this is now under examination).

Phenobarbital is scarcely used today in industrialised countries, mainly because of its sedative effects. It is less teratogenic than valproate and it is still a useful AED in countries with poor resources.

Gabapentin is of very low efficacy, is associated with weight gain and has still unexplored effects in pregnancy.

Topiramate has high efficacy, but is seriously hindered by numerous ADRs that may also affect the foetus and the newborn of women with epilepsy.

> *Therefore, the first choice in the treatment of women with focal seizures is between carbamazepine, lamotrigine, levetiracetam and oxcarbazepine.*

Carbamazepine still remains one of the most effective AEDs and appears to be relatively safe for women. It is an enzyme inducer, but its reputation as a pregnancy category D drug has been partly restored in recent evidence-based studies (Table 2.2).

Oxcarbazepine is still difficult to assess precisely and to ascertain whether it is better than carbamazepine as initially promoted. Its decrease plasma concentration during pregnancy has been associated with seizure deterioration.

Lamotrigine has been extensively promoted as the most women-friendly AED and the number of prescriptions for women is rising. However, recent evidence indicates that its use is associated with significant problems, including interactions with hormonal contraception and pregnancy that may cause an increase of seizures or toxicity, and its teratogenic potential has not been yet elucidated, with some class 1 and 2 studies reporting a dose-related effect on MCM.[176] Adjunctive treatment with lamotrigine and valproate is one of the most teratogenic combinations.

Levetiracetam is more effective than lamotrigine and class 1 studies indicate that it has very low teratogenic potential (Table 2.2), but this needs to be replicated when a larger number of women are recruited in the pregnancy registries. It is unknown whether its reduced plasma concentration during pregnancy is of clinical significance (i.e. whether levetiracetam, like lamotrigine and oxcarbazepine, may be associated with seizure deterioration in women during pregnancy).

Commencing AED therapy in women of childbearing age with newly diagnosed generalised epilepsy

Valproate is unequivocally the most effective AED in generalised epilepsies, so what is the best option for women of childbearing age for whom valproate is now practically impossible to prescribe? In the past, and before the introduction of newer broad-spectrum AEDs, when valproate was the only option for the treatment of generalised epilepsies, we used to inform the patient thoroughly about the pros (best option for protection against generalised seizures) and cons (worse option with regard to teratogenicity and spina bifida) of this drug. We now have the advantage of having lamotrigine and levetiracetam as other options, but we have to detail the pros and cons of each. Lamotrigine is not as innocuous in women as we initially thought; GTCS may worsen during pregnancy in women on this drug and it often aggravates myoclonic jerks. Currently, levetiracetam appears to be the best substitute for valproate in the treatment of women with generalised epilepsies, though the verdict is still open.

Preconception

The preconception period is important to establish optimal seizure control with the most appropriate pregnancy-friendly AED.

Optimisation of AED therapy involves:
(a) re-evaluation of the diagnosis using the same steps listed on pages 5–10: are the paroxysmal events epileptic; what type of seizures are they; what causes them; and which epileptic syndrome is it?
(b) assessment of the frequency and severity of seizures before and after AED therapy, as well as possible precipitating factors and circadian distribution
(c) recording the course and outcome of previous pregnancies if there were any
(d) consideration of whether current AED therapy is optimal for the patient and the infant, or whether changes are needed, which is probably the case in the women taking valproate and/or polytherapy.

Some women are determined to avoid any AED-induced risks to their babies and stop taking their medication from the time that they prepare to conceive. Withdrawal of AED before pregnancy might be considered if the woman:

- is free of seizures for more than 2 years, though relapse is possible particularly in syndromes such as JME, which often relapse on AED withdrawal
- does not have GTCS or seizures that may result in injury, though these may appear in well-controlled syndromes after AED withdrawal
- the potential consequences of seizure recurrence is thoroughly informed of.

For women in whom seizures are controlled by monotherapy with any AED other than valproate, there is probably no need for any change. The worse possible scenario for the physician is having to make appropriate decisions for women with generalised epilepsies who are controlled on valproate. This is because of the uncertainties with regard to possible relapses that may occur when another AED is substituted, which may not be a problem for women with focal epilepsies as explained above. In generalised epilepsies, the attempt to switch to levetiracetam (or as a second option to lamotrigine) should be made with caution, because of the possibility of seizure recurrence, particularly with lamotrigine. Women with JME should be informed that lamotrigine is not as effective as valproate and levetiracetam and also carries an increased risk of aggravating myoclonic seizures. If valproate is to be maintained, attempts should be made to reduce it to a minimal dosage, possibly divided into 3–4 daily doses.

Women who are controlled on AED polytherapy should, if possible, be converted to monotherapy or to two AEDs by slowly withdrawing the AEDs that are undesirable in women. Again the patient should be warned of the possibility of relapse.

For women who are not controlled on AEDs, the situation is exactly the same as for any other patient who seeks control of seizures, but women-friendly AEDs should be given priority.

Folic acid should be prescribed before and throughout the first trimester.

It is common for women to become pregnant while taking AEDs without preconception advice.

The role of the physician is to assess the situation regarding seizures and ADRs, inform the patient and request appropriate tests for the mother and foetus. The possible teratogenic effect of AEDs has been exerted by the end of the first trimester, but cognitive or other effects on the fetus may occur throughout the pregnancy.

Any changes to AED treatment should be made before conception.

Follow-up of women with epilepsy during pregnancy and after delivery should be meticulous and requires good communication between the treating physician, the obstetrician and midwife in addition to expert prenatal screening and TDM of AEDs that are affected by pregnancy and carry the possibility of seizure relapse, such as lamotrigine and oxcarbazepine. Almost all neural tube defects can be detected by week 20 using high resolution ultrasonography. Routine screening for α-fetoprotein in amniotic fluid probably provides little additional value.[221] Most of the other MCM can also be diagnosed by ultrasonography, but their severity is difficult to assess prenatally.

> *Women with epileptic seizures should be reassured that they can have happy families with healthy children like any other woman. Their pregnancies may carry some definite risks, but these are small and can be minimised through proper management before, during and after pregnancy.*

Principles of Management in the Elderly with Epileptic Seizures

3

In the last decade, increasing attention has been paid to improving the management of the elderly with epileptic seizures,who have many unmet needs. [222-226]

(a) The global elderly population is constantly increasing and the average life expectancy is 78–82 years in the USA, European Union, Japan and Australia (with women living 2–3 years longer than men); one-tenth of the world population is over the age of 60 years.

(b) The prevalence and incidence of epilepsy increases sharply in this population (Figure 1.4)[225] and epilepsy is the third most common neurological condition after cerebrovascular disease and dementia.

(c) Diagnosis is challenging, because co-morbid disorders may imitate epilepsy.

(d) When choosing an AED, it is important to consider the significant pharmacokinetic changes that occur in the elderly as well as co-medications for other co-morbidities.

(e) The elderly are particularly vulnerable to ADRs of AEDs, which are often poorly communicated and assessed.

The proceedings of an expert International Geriatric Epilepsy Symposium were recently published in a supplement of *Epilepsy Research* (2006).[227]

The increase in the incidence and prevalence of epileptic seizures in the elderly is due to co-morbid disorders. Cerebrovasular disease prevails, (30–40%) followed by metabolic disturbances, trauma, central nervous system infections, space-occupying lesions and others.[225] Acute (provoked, occasional) symptomatic seizures are common. Conversely, elderly patients with pre-existing epilepsy often experience an improvement in or remission of seizures, as for example with many IGEs such as JME.

Focal seizures are the predominant or exclusive seizure type with or without secondarily GTCS in the elderly. Extratemporal focal seizures are more common than in younger patients. GTCS are also predominantly of focal onset.

Difficulties in diagnosing epileptic seizures in the elderly

Epileptic seizures are often unrecognised or mistaken for non-epileptic paroxysmal events in the elderly.[226] Their manifestations commonly mimic the symptoms of cerebrovascular disease or are considered 'natural' phenomena associated with the ageing process. An epileptic fall, for example, is more likely to be attributed to cerebral ischaemia, loss of balance or be accidental. An epileptic complex focal seizure with impairment of consciousness is more likely to be considered cerebrovascular or an event of an age-related memory deficit. The diagnostic difficulties are even greater when the patient also has symptoms of cerebrovacular disease, dementia or cardiac problems.

Social isolation, lack of witnesses and the difficulty or inability of the elderly to describe their symptoms are factors that are compounded in the misdiagnosis of epileptic seizures in the elderly.

Frequency of seizures and their severity in the elderly

It is generally accepted that seizures in the elderly are usually infrequent and easily controlled with AEDs, which is also my experience. This view has been validated in a recent study of newly diagnosed elderly patients with epilepsy, which showed that 84% of patients achieved seizure freedom with proper management and that this was statistically significant when compared with newly diagnosed younger populations (p < 0.001).[228] Further, in RCTs a patient with a "minimum of one seizure (>60% with two or more seizures) during the 3 months preceding enrolment is considered representative of patients with new-onset geriatric epilepsy".[44]

The majority of focal seizures may not be severe, but the effect of convulsive seizures when they occur in an already vulnerable and sometimes disabled elderly individual may be devastating. Post-ictal confusion may be particularly severe and lengthy (lasting for days) compared with that in younger individuals. The prevalence of status epilepticus is almost twice that in the general population and the mortality (38–50%) is the highest of any age group.[223] Convulsive status epilepticus commonly manifests in the acute state of a cerebral insult (see acute symptomatic seizures). Focal symptomatic non-convulsive status epilepticus and less commonly absence status epilepticus are widely misdiagnosed in any age group, but probably more so in the elderly even if it is protracted for days.[229] Absence status epilepticus in the elderly mainly occurs de novo after benzodiazepine withdrawal.[230]

EEG and other investigative procedures in the elderly

Requests for investigative procedures in the elderly should be limited to those that are absolutely necessary. Otherwise, the patient may suffer unnecessary discomfort. False-positive EEG and brain MRI results are common.

Elderly patients require the same care and diagnostic precision as younger people. Therefore, the diagnostic procedures are universally the same. However, considering that the elderly are often fragile, diagnostic procedures should be limited to those that are absolutely necessary.

Useful clinical advice

The overenthusiastic approach – "Let us do this test as well not to miss that remote possibility" – is discouraged, particularly as 'this test' may be invasive, extremely unpleasant and intolerable to an elderly person in addition to the extra burden of transport from home to the hospital.

Diagnosis should mainly rely on clinical assessment. Blood tests often identify problems such as metabolic or drug-induced toxicity without the need for further tests.

EEG and brain imaging, the two main investigative procedures in the epilepsies, are significantly affected by age and therefore false-positive results are high in the elderly. EEG background abnormalities are common in the elderly and this is the rule rather than exception, particularly in those with cerebrovasular disease and dementia, and those taking psychotropic drugs. Sharp waves and other paroxysmal or focal abnormalities are not of the same diagnostic significance as in younger populations. It is because of all these factors that my EEG reports for an elderly person referred for possible epileptic seizures include the following comment:

> "The EEG is abnormal. However, the reason for this and its clinical significance are uncertain. It cannot be taken as evidence for or against epileptic seizures. Such EEG abnormalities in patients of this age are common. Conversely, elderly patients with definite epileptic seizures may not have the classical spikes or other EEG markers of epileptogenicity that we assess in younger people."

However, rarely EEG may capture ictal events and EEG is of the utmost importance in patients with suspected non-convulsive status epilepticus.

Physiological and other changes in the elderly that may affect AEDs

AED pharmacokinetics may be affected in the elderly, because ageing is associated with significant physiological and other changes.[78,222,231]

(a) Bioavailability may be reduced because of a decline in the ability to absorb the drug; this may particularly affect gabapentin.

(b) Free fractions of protein-bound AEDs may increase significantly (which may not show in TDM) and cause toxicity.

(c) Plasma levels of enzyme-inducing AEDs (Table 1.6) may increase significantly and the elimination half-life may be prolonged because of the declining efficiency of the P450 system, decreasing liver volume and slowing of blood flow. Hepatic glucoronidation is less affected.

(d) For most AEDs that are metabolised and excreted by the kidneys, the clearance of unbound drug is decreased by an average of 20–40% in the elderly.[231]

(e) Plasma levels of AEDs that are primarily excreted in the urine (Table 1.8) may increase significantly because of declining renal function and lower glomerular filtration rate.

The elderly usually have a narrower therapeutic window; that is, the maximum tolerated AED concentration is closer to the lowest therapeutic concentration.[232]

Principles of AED treatment in the elderly

AED treatment of the elderly is significantly different than that of younger adult patients. Elderly patients are more likely to suffer from drug-induced disease than to derive any benefits from ill-advised AED prescribing.

Seizures are predominantly focal with or without secondarily GTCS. Therefore, the choice is between AEDs listed in Table 3.1 that are licensed for the treatment of focal epilepsies in adults and the elderly. Broad-spectrum AEDs are needed for the few cases of elderly patients with generalised or a mixed type of seizures.

Elderly patients respond well to lower doses and they are particularly sensitive to ADRs. Co-morbidity and co-medication is prominent. Therefore, 'start very low and go very slow' and other procedures of titration detailed in the useful clinical notes are particularly valuable in the AED treatment of the elderly. Small doses, usually half the recommended initial and maintenance dose for adults, may often be therapeutic. ADRs that are common, often severe and underdiagnosed or misdiagnosed may be avoidable by selecting the right AED (Table 3.1) and using very small doses.

Excellent pharmacokinetics, minimal interactions with other drugs and negligible ADRs are the optimal factors in choosing an AED for the elderly (Table 3.1). An ability to achieve a therapeutic effect without titration, parenteral formulations and ease of swallowing are also desirable attributes.[234]

Polypharmacy is discouraged because ADRs and drug–drug interactions are more likely than true seizure benefit. Patients starting treatment two or more years after their first seizure are less likely to achieve seizure control than patients in whom treatment was initiated earlier.[228]

In RCTs in adults (including a variable number of the elderly), all AEDs licensed for monotherapy for focal epilepsy (Table 3.1) have shown approximately equal efficacy. In the elderly, there is a paucity of class I and class II RCTs.[44,235] Only gabapentin[236] and lamotrigine[233,236,237] have been adequately tested in face-to-face comparisons with carbamazepine. Although these drugs had similar efficacy, carbamazepine was less well tolerated. Whether the results would be different at different doses, different titration scheme and different methodology is the usual question in these RCTs.

Significant clinical note

The key recommendation in the treatment of the elderly is to avoid AEDs with:

- ADRs that may cause more harm (cognitive impairment, confusion, fractures, falls, cardiac abnormalities, ataxia, allergies) than good (seizure improvement is often achieved with small doses of relatively ADR-free AEDs)

- drug–drug interactions (such as with enzyme-inducers) that may adversely affect concomitant medications and vice versa

Small doses, usually half the recommended initial and maintenance dose for adults, may often be therapeutic.

Little information is available on the use and the effect of AEDs in elderly who have co-morbid cardiological disorders.

AEDs licensed for monotherapy in focal seizures with and without secondarily GTCSs: comparison of priorities that are important in the treatment of elderly with epilepsy*

	Toler-ability	Pharma-cokinetics (% of perfect score)[†]	Significant drug–drug interactions	Titration	Need for laboratory tests[‡]	Parenteral formulation
Carba-mazepine	Medium	Inferior (50)	Yes	Slow	Maximal (1 and 2)	No
Lamot-rigine	Excellent	Moderate (73)	Yes	Very slow	Maximal (1 and 2)	No
Levetira-cetam	Excellent	Superior (96)	Not clinically significant	Fast	Minimal	Yes
Gabap-entin	Excellent	Superior (89)	Not clinically significant	Fast	Minimal	No
Oxcar-bazepine	Medium	Moderate (77)	Yes	Slow	Maximal (1 and 2)	No
Pheno-barbital	Poor	Inferior (57)	Yes	Slow	Maximal (1 and 2)	Yes
Phenytoin	Poor	Inferior (50)	Yes	Slow	Maximal (1 and 2)	Yes
Topir-amate	Poor	Moderate (79)	Yes	Very slow	Maximal (1 and 2)	No
Valproate	Poor	Inferior (52)	Yes	Slow	Maximal (1)	Yes

Table 3.1 Desirable properties are in red. *All AEDs in this table are lisenced for elderly patients in monotherapy of focal seizures. In RCTs, none of the newer AEDs showed better efficacy than carbamazepine but they were better tolerated; gabapentin has shown worse efficacy in clinical practice. For more information, see summary of product characteristics and Table 1.2. [†]The % of perfect score is based on a customised rating system of 16 parameters to evaluate the pharmacokinetic profile of AEDs developed by Patsalos.[233] [‡](1) Monitoring for adverse drug reactions; (2) therapeutic drug monitoring.

Surgery for Epilepsies

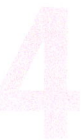

The surgical treatment of drug-resistant epilepsy has become increasingly more valuable and often life-saving due to major advances in structural and functional neuroimaging, EEG monitoring and surgical techniques. The outcome from current surgical methods has improved dramatically.[238–240] Paediatric surgical outcomes have become similar to those reported for adults.[241,242]

Early surgical intervention, when successful, might also prevent or reverse the disabling psychosocial consequences of uncontrolled seizures during critical periods of development.

Despite this progress, surgery in epilepsies is underused and referrals are often delayed or not made.[238,243] The reasons for this delay include the fears of the patients and physicians about surgery and undue reliance on newer AEDs and vagus nerve stimulation (VNS) in patients who had failed to respond to appropriate medical treatment for years.

The applications and outcomes of surgical interventions in certain types of intractable seizures and epileptic syndromes are detailed in the relevant chapters of this book. This section refers to general aspects of surgery in epilepsies. This topic has recently been covered in over 300 pages in one of the best books on the treatment of epilepsies – *The Treatment of Epilepsy*.[244]

Surgical treatment for epilepsy need not be a last resort.

Often, successful surgery, particularly in children, is too late to reverse the crippling psychological and social consequences of repeated epileptic seizures during developmental ages that are critical for the acquisition of interpersonal and vocational skills. These patients, even if they remain seizure-free, are permanently disabled.[238]

A new classification of outcome with respect to epileptic seizures following epilepsy surgery has been issued by the ILAE Commission.[245] More recently, the ILAE Subcommission for Paediatric Epilepsy Surgery has published a consensus statement on the unique features of paediatric epilepsy patients that justifies dedicated resources and specialty paediatric surgical centres; guidelines for physicians for when to initiate the referral process for children with refractory epilepsy; and recommendations on presurgical evaluation and post-operative assessments.[242]

C.P. Panayiotopoulos, *Principles of Therapy in the Epilepsies*,
© Springer-Verlag London Limited 2011

Criteria for surgical referral

A candidate for epilepsy surgery must:

- have failed to attain adequate seizure control with adequate trials of antiepileptic drugs (drug-resistant epilepsy) or suffer from surgically remediable syndromes
- have a reasonable chance of benefitting from surgery.

Paediatric referrals differ from that of adults in two important respects.[242] First, seizures in childhood may be associated with developmental arrest or regression, especially in children younger than 2 years. Second, focal epilepsy in childhood is often associated with age-specific aetiologies such as Sturge–Weber or Landau–Kleffner syndrome, hemispheric and other malformations of brain development. Currently, no pre-operative clinical variables predict seizure outcome in the paediatric surgical population.[242] Developmental delay or psychiatric morbidity are not contraindicated for paediatric epilepsy surgery.[242]

Drug-resistant epilepsy for the purposes of surgical referral

Intractable epilepsy is defined in many ways.[240,247] Drug-resistant epilepsy for the purposes of surgical referral is defined by an inadequate response to a minimum of two first-line AEDs, either as monotherapy or in combination, as appropriate to the epileptic syndrome. The recommended duration is at least 2 years of treatment in adults; however, this may be too long for children when considering the consequences of continuing seizures on their development.

The concept of surgically remediable epileptic syndromes

This concept was introduced in order to promote early surgical intervention for certain forms of epilepsy with well-defined pathophysiological substrates that are known to have a poor prognosis after failure of a few AEDs and an excellent surgical prognosis.[248]

The following are the main surgically remediable epileptic syndromes:

- mesial temporal lobe epilepsy with hippocampal sclerosis (hippocampal epilepsy)
- certain temporal or extratemporal neocortical symptomatic focal syndromes with discrete easily resectable structural lesions
- epilepsies of infants and small children that can be treated with hemispherectomy.

Strategy of a surgical work-up

A pre-surgical evaluation and surgery should be carried out in specialised centres for these procedures, which usually differ in children and adults.

A pre-surgical evaluation of candidates for surgery includes:

- an accurate diagnosis based on a meticulous ictal and inter-ictal clinical history
- neuroradiological investigations and particularly high-resolution MRI, often supplemented with functional brain imaging
- neurophysiological identification of the epileptogenic brain region
- neuropsychological evaluation to reveal possible cognitive and linguistic deficits and to predict the effect of cortical resection
- quality of life and psychiatric assessment.

Subsequently, a decision is taken on the most appropriate surgical strategy and the potential outcome is estimated.

Resective surgery is most likely to be successful if the findings from different modalities are concordant with regard to epileptogenic localisation.

Useful warning to patients

Patients referred to specialised surgery centres should be warned of the following:
- waiting lists may be long
- evaluation procedures are often lengthy, lasting for months
- they may not be suitable for surgery.

Types of surgical procedures

Surgery can be one of two types:

1. *Curative (or definitive),* aiming at suppression of the epileptogenic focus through a resective or disconnective surgical procedure.

2. *Palliative (or functional)* with the purpose of reducing the intensity and/ or the frequency of a certain seizure type (callosotomy and multiple subpial transections).

Curative (definitive) surgery

Curative surgery physically removes seizure-producing brain tissue and carries a significant chance of producing complete, or at least 90%, improvement in seizures.

Focal resective procedure (lesionectomy)

This is the most common, important and rewarding of all surgical treatments for focal epilepsies. The aim is to resect the total irritative zone to a sufficient extent to lead to the elimination of seizures.

Hippocampal epilepsy benefits most from this procedure. A class 1 RCT of surgery for hippocampal epilepsy found that 64% of those who received surgery were free of disabling seizures compared with 8% in the group randomised to continued AED medical therapy. Quality of life and social function significantly improved in the patients who were operated on; morbidity was infrequent and there was no mortality.[238]

Complications are rare, probably less than 1% or 2% overall, and vary with the experience of the surgical team rather than the procedure.

Other temporal and extratemporal epilepsies benefit from resective surgery, which also produces excellent results (see the surgical treatment of relevant focal epilepsies). In these cases the discreteness of the lesion and its relationship to eloquent cortical areas are major determinants of surgical management and outcome.

Often surgical problems may be difficult, needing complex investigative tools such as functional MRI (fMRI), magnetoencephalography (MEG), invasive recording and operating with neuronavigation and possibly intra-operative MRI.[239] The most difficult part is to define exactly the whole area of the irritative brain tissue, because this frequently extends beyond the structural lesion visualised on neuroimaging or the epileptogenic cortical area generating inter-ictal spikes. Where there is no discrete lesion (cryptogenic focal epilepsies), fMRI and both acute and chronic electrophysiological recordings may be helpful in determining the extent of the resection.

In hypothalamic epilepsy, resective epilepsy has now improved, but it still has high risks. Several different approaches have been used successfully, but their relative efficacy and safety have not yet been established.[242]

Cerebral hemispherectomy

Cerebral hemispherectomy for intractable seizures has evolved over the past 50 years and current operations focus less on brain resection and more on disconnection. The main indications are drug-resistant seizures secondary to gross unilateral hemispherical pathology with severe contralateral (to the lesion) neurological deficit, including hemianopia. Common conditions for which hemispherectomy is recommended include Kozhevnikov–Rasmussen syndrome, hemiconvulsion–hemiplegia syndrome, hemimegaloencephaly and miscellaneous hemispherical residual atrophic or other lesions, including Sturge–Weber disease.[242] The structural and functional integrity of the other hemisphere should be appropriately verified.

Seizure outcome is excellent with three-quarters (58–78%) of patients becoming seizure free, and it is generally perceived that behaviour and intellectual performance improve in these patients. Outcome is related to the completeness of disconnection and less so to aetiology, although those with malformations of cortical development appear to do worse than others. The surgical mortality rate is low (0–6%).

Palliative (functional) surgery[249]

Palliative surgery is designed to improve seizures by modification of the neuronal pathways responsible for their generation and spreading. Its purpose is to reduce the intensity and frequency of certain seizure types. It rarely (3–5%) results in freedom from seizures.

Corpus callosotomy

Corpus callosotomy, surgical division of the corpus callosum, is the only procedure for devastating atonic seizures with traumatic falls (atonic drop attacks) of epileptic encephalopathies. A favourable outcome, from a greater than 50% reduction to occasional complete cessation of these seizures, is obtained in 60–80% of patients. Improvements (40–80%) have also been reported in symptomatic tonic seizures and less often secondary GTCSs according to the extension of the section. These are cases of symptomatic secondarily generalised epilepsy with EEG bifrontal epileptic foci and secondary bilateral synchrony. Global behavioural and intellectual improvement may occur, particularly if surgery is performed early. Other types of seizures are not indicated for callosotomy, even though some improvement may be observed.

Despite improvements and modifications of corpus callosotomy with sequential radiofrequency lesions and stereotactic radiosurgery, morbidity is relatively high and there is a tendency for seizures to return after 2 years. More severe focal seizures may occur postoperatively.

Multiple subpial transections

Multiple subpial transection is an ingenious surgical technique invented by Morrell[250,251] for drug-resistant focal epilepsies involving eloquent motor-, sensory- or language-important cortex and Landau–Kleffner syndrome. This technique eliminates the capacity of cortical tissue to generate seizures while preserving the normal cortical physiological function.

The rationale of the technique is based on the observation that horizontal fibres of the cortex facilitate the propagation of epileptic discharge, whereas the vertical fibres subserve function. Thus, surgical division of the tangential fibres at regular intervals in a cortical epileptogenic area would permanently disrupt side-to-side, intracortical, synchronising, neuronal networks and curtail the epileptic discharges. Function is preserved because these right-angle cuts to the pial surface should not disrupt cortex–subcortical, input–output interactions.

The success of the technique depends on selection of cases with severe epileptogenic abnormality that can be demonstrated to be unilateral in origin despite a bilateral electrographic manifestation.

Vagus Nerve Stimulation

Vagus nerve stimulation (VNS)[252–256] is an invasive non-pharmacological treatment licensed for use as an adjunctive therapy in reducing the frequency of seizures in adults and adolescents over 12 years of age with focal seizures which are resistant to AEDs. It is also licensed for treatment-resistant depression.

Efficacy

Systematic reviews of the current evidence for the effects of VNS in drug-resistant focal seizures have concluded that this is an effective and well-tolerated treatment.[253] In general, a third of the patients show more than 50% reduction in seizure frequency (but seizure freedom is conspicuously extremely rare), a third show a 30–50% seizure reduction and a third show no response.[257] Concomitant AEDs may be reduced, but I am not aware of any reports of patients where all drugs were withdrawn, thereby using VNS as monotherapy. All patients stay on at least one medication in addition to the VNS. Improvements in various quality-of-life measurements during treatment with VNS have been reported.[258] In practice VNS has been used for a variety of drug-resistant epilepsies, including young children with epileptic encephalopathies, but the results are often conflicting, ranging from good to no effect. In one of the best-controlled studies, 16 children with epileptic encephalopathies were treated with VNS and followed up for 3 years.[259] There were significant fluctuations in effectiveness, but at the end of the study all children were no better than their pre-VNS baselines with regard to seizures and parameters of quality of life.[260] This contradicts the idea based on anecdotal evidence that seizure control and quality-of-life benefits with VNS treatment increase over time, and that improvement may not be immediate but happens over 18–24 months of treatment.

Adverse reactions

Surgery-related complications: infection (3%), which may demand the removal of the device (1%), vocal cord dysfunction (hoarseness and dysphagia) (1%), facial nerve palsy, Horner's syndrome, bradycardia and, exceptionally, asystole (0.1%), wound haematoma and lead breakage (0.1%), and aesthetic complications from the incisions (prevalence unknown).

Perioperative adverse reactions: pain (29%), coughing (14%), voice alteration (13%), chest pain (12%) and nausea (10%).

During treatment: hoarseness (37%), throat pain (11%), coughing (7%), dyspnoea (6%), paraesthesiae (6%), muscle pain (6%) and discomfort in the face or neck when the stimulator is activated. All are related to the intensity of stimulation, can often be reduced by adjusting the generator's programme and may habituate in most individuals.

There are no apparent effects of VNS on vagally medicated visceral functions or AED plasma concentrations. No adverse cognitive or systemic effects are reported with the use of the implanted vagus nerve stimulator.

Technical aspects

The VNS device (manufactured by Cyberonics, Inc.; www.cyberonics.com) consists of a small, battery-powered, electrical pulse generator implanted under the skin of the left chest. This is linked to the stimulating spring-shaped electrodes that are wrapped around the main trunk of the left vagus nerve via an under-the-skin insulated cable.

The pulse generator is individually programmed to stimulate the left vagus nerve automatically at varying frequencies, typically for 30 s every 5 min, through a computer and a hand-held 'wand'. The frequency is adjusted to the patient's needs.

The treating physician makes readjustments to the programming and stimulus output.

In addition, the patient or carer can activate extra-stimulation at pre-programmed settings through a magnet passed over the generator. This is to shorten or terminate a seizure as soon as possible after its onset. Keeping the magnet over the generator turns off the stimulation.

Surgical procedure and cost

The implantation of the VNS therapeutic device is a surgical procedure requiring general anaesthesia. It is usually performed by an experienced neurosurgeon and it takes approximately 1 or 2 hours. The generator is inserted in the hollow below the clavicle through an incision in the left axilla. The electrodes are inserted through an incision in the left side of the neck. Patients usually go home the same day that the VNS device is implanted.

The cost is substantial. In addition to the cost of hospitalisation and the operation, the cost of the VNS device is approximately US$15,600. The battery lasts between 3 and 5 years (10 years in the current versions) and is replaced by a small operation under local anaesthesia. A replacement VNS device with new battery is US$11,600.

What is the place of VNS in the treatment of epilepsies?

Reports fulfilling the requirements of evidence-based medicine conclude that VNS is effective in drug-resistant focal epilepsies (when multiple polytherapy has failed) and may improve the quality of life. Similar studies on the effect of VNS in epileptic encephalopathies have been disappointing.

Reports from uncontrolled studies, case reports and their reviews are also in favour of VNS in a number of drug-resistant epileptic disorders including epileptic en cephalopathies. Of 129 children from 12 centres in the USA, 72 had a 12-month follow-up or more, with all 129 having follow-up for at least 6 months. Overall, only one child was seizure free and 43% demonstrated greater than 50% improvement, but 43% had no change in seizure frequency.[242] Some data were promising with regard to drop attacks, but the role of VNS versus callosotomy requires further evaluation.[242]

In clinical practice, the opinion of expert paediatric and adult epileptologists that I share is far less enthusiastic:

A few patients may improve.

Some patients have less hospital admissions.

I would try it in patients who had failed AED therapy and are not suitable for operation but I would not give great hopes to the patients who may also have to meet a significant cost.

An expensive and useless exercise in epileptic encephalopathies.

The truth may be somewhere between these views.

VNS may have a place in drug-resistant epilepsies that are not amicable to surgery.

In a recent study, concurrent (ketogenic or modified Atkins) diet and VNS treatment for medically drug-resistant childhood epilepsy appeared synergistic and yielded rapid 'benefits'.[261]

Useful note

Environmental precautions for those treated with VNS

Strong magnets such as those used in MRI, loudspeakers and hair clippers may interfere with the stimulator or the electrode leads. Body MRI is contraindicated, whereas head MRI should be done with only transmit-and-receive head coils. In general, 'avoid areas where pacemaker warning signs are posted'.

The magnet provided for manual stimulation may damage credit cards, mobile phones, computer disks, televisions and other items affected by strong magnetic fields. Care should be taken to store the magnet away from these types of equipment.

Ketogenic Diet

The ketogenic diet[262-272] is undergoing a mini-renaissance in drug-resistant childhood epilepsies and particularly epileptic encephalopathies.

The ketogenic diet and related dietary treatments have been recently reviewed.[273]

Indications and efficacy

Large observational studies, some prospective, and one RCT,[272] are consistent in showing that the ketogenic diet is a relatively safe and effective treatment in infants and children with drug-resistant epilepsies. The diet is particularly effective for epileptic spasms and epilepsies with myoclonic seizures. Overall, estimates indicate that complete cessation of all seizures occurs in 16% of patients, a greater than 90% reduction in seizures occurs in 32%, and a greater than 50% reduction in seizures occurs in 56%.[262] Half the children will continue on the diet for at least 1 year; 40–50% of those starting the diet will have a greater than 50% reduction in seizures after 12 months. Most parents also report improvements in their child's behaviour and function, particularly with respect to attention/alertness, activity level and socialisation.[263] A concomitant reduction in AEDs is often possible. The ketogenic diet is first-line therapy for the treatment of seizures due to glucose transporter protein deficiency.[274]

Rationale and types of ketogenic diet

The ketogenic diet as an effective treatment of drug-resistant epilepsies was introduced in 1921 as a way of duplicating and prolonging the beneficial effects that fasting appeared to have on seizure control. Hence, this diet mimics the changes of starvation. Neurones use ketone bodies rather than glucose as a metabolic substrate. The mechanism of action of the diet remains unknown, and it is difficult to assess which biochemical parameters should be monitored as adjustments are made to the diet. It has been suggested that chronic ketosis may control seizures by increasing the cerebral energy reserves in the brain, thus promoting neuronal stability.

The ketogenic diet is a high-fat, low-carbohydrate, low-protein regimen. The ketogenic ratio (fat:carbohydrate plus protein) ranges from 2:1 to a maximum of 5:1. The constituents are customised to meet the patient's needs and preferences. The diet is a radical medical therapy and nutritional well-being is a constant concern. The diet is usually started as an inpatient. It should be initiated, supervised and monitored by a nutrition support team who also instruct family members on the maintenance of the diet at home. Traditionally, children starting on the ketogenic diet were made to fast for 1 or 2 days until ketosis was seen. They were then started on a third of the calories for 24 hours, then two-thirds of the calories for the next 24 hours, and finally were advanced to a full diet. This fasting period is often a difficult time for young children and their families, and is probably not needed.[275]

The Atkins diet

The popular Atkins diet has recently been used in the treatment of epileptic encephalopathies as a less restrictive alternative therapy to the ketogenic diet.[276–278]

Adverse effects of the ketogenic diet

The ketogenic diet is generally well tolerated and over 94% of patients have maintained appropriate growth parameters.[8] Nephrolithiasis has been reported in 5–8% of children. Other adverse events have included a reduced quantity of bone mass (requiring vitamin D supplementation), gastritis, ulcerative colitis, alteration of mentation and hyperlipidaemia. Altered concentrations of AEDs may cause toxicity. Carbonic anhydrase inhibitors (Table 1.7) should be avoided. When possible, valproate should also be avoided. The diet may be lethal for patients with rare disorders of cerebral energy metabolisms such as pyruvate carboxylase deficiency.

Corticosteroids in the Treatment of Childhood Epilepsies

Corticosteroids are sometimes used to treat severe forms of childhood epilepsies in an attempt to reduce seizures and improve behaviour, cognitive function, motor function or any combination of these.[279–281] Their mechanism of action is unknown, the evidence base for their use is weak (except for epileptic spasms) and their potential ADRs are considerable. Corticosteroid treatment is clinically beneficial only in the treatment of West syndrome, epileptic encephalopathy with continuous spike-and-wave during sleep (which includes Landau–Kleffner syndrome) and possibly Kozhevnikov–Rasmussen syndrome. For all other drug-resistant epilepsies, corticosteroid treatment is usually a somewhat desperate move when other therapies have failed, and it is usually administered during periods when control of seizures is particularly problematic. Corticosteroids are also sometimes used for children with protracted and frequent episodes of status epilepticus, mainly in epileptic encephalopathies. It is important to clearly define the purpose of such treatment before its start.

Preparation, doses and regimens of corticosteroids

A variety of preparations are available. Oral prednisone or intramuscular adrenocorticotrophic hormone (ACTH) are the most commonly used.

With ACTH, dose regimens vary from 20 IU/day to 150 IU/m^2 per day. Efficacy and tolerability of natural ACTH is considered to be better than its synthetic analogue tetracosactide (tetracosactrin).

Prednisone is usually given at 1, 2 or 3 mg/kg per day. Other corticosteroids include oral hydrocortisone, betamethasone and dexamethasone (sometimes also intravenously).

Corticosteroids have been given in short courses of a few weeks or longer courses lasting many months. Both non-tapered and tapered regimens have been advocated.

Adverse effects and monitoring of corticosteroid treatment

Corticosteroid treatment is associated with significant adverse effects, particularly when used at high doses and over prolonged periods. Some of these may be fatal. Of more concern are electrolyte disturbances, glucose intolerance, hypertension, increased susceptibility to infections, particularly to certain viral infections such as varicella, and osteoporosis, myopathy and cardiomyopathy. Treatment is also associated with an increase in the ventricular and extra-axial cerebrospinal fluid spaces, which is apparent on brain imaging and usually reversible.

References

1. Bodde NM, Brooks JL, Baker GA, Boon PA, Hendriksen JG, Mulder OG et al. Psychogenic non-epileptic seizures--diagnostic issues: a critical review. Clin Neurol Neurosurg 2009;111:1–9.
2. National Institute for Health and Clinical Excellence (NICE). The epilepsies: the diagnosis and management of the epilepsies in adults and children in primary and secondary care. www.nice org uk/page aspx?o=227586, 2004. Last accessed 27 September 2009.
3. Tegretol® (carbamazepine). Summary of product characteristics. Novartis Pharmaceuticals UK Ltd, 2009.
4. Frisium® (clobazam). Summary of product characteristics. Sanofi-aventis, 2009.
5. Rivotril® (clonazepam). Summary of product characteristics. Roche Products Ltd, 2009.
6. Zarontin® (ethosuximide). Summary of product characteristics. Pfizer Ltd, 2009.
7. Neurontin® (gabapentin). Summary of product characteristics. Pfizer Ltd, 2009.
8. Vimpat® (lacosamide). Summary of product characteristics. UCB Pharma Ltd, 2009.
9. Lamictal® (lamotrigine). Summary of product characteristics. GlaxoSmithKline UK Ltd, 2009.
10. Keppra® (levetiracetam). Summary of product characteristics. UCB Pharma Ltd, 2009.
11. Trileptal® (oxcarbazepine). Summary of product characteristics. Novartis Pharmaceuticals UK Ltd, 2009.
12. Phenobarbital. Summary of product characteristics. Actavis UK Ltd, 2009.
13. Epanutin® (phenytoin). Summary of product characteristics. Pfizer Ltd, 2009.
14. Lyrica® (pregabalin). Summary of product characteristics. Pfizer Ltd, 2009.
15. Gabitril® (tiagabine). Summary of product characteristics. Cephalon (UK) Ltd, 2009.
16. Topamax® (topiramate). Summary of product characteristics. Janssen-Cilag Ltd, 2009.
17. Epilim® (sodium valproate). Summary of product characteristics. Sanofi-aventis, 2009.
18. Sabril® (vigabatrin). Summary of product characteristics. Sanofi-aventis, 2009.
19. Zonegran® (zonisamide). Summary of product characteristics. Eisai Ltd, 2009.
20. Panayiotopoulos CP, Chroni E, Daskalopoulos C, Baker A, Rowlinson S, Walsh P. Typical absence seizures in adults: clinical, EEG, video-EEG findings and diagnostic/syndromic considerations. J Neurol Neurosurg Psychiatr 1992;55:1002–8.
21. Liporace JD, Sperling MR, Dichter MA. Absence seizures and carbamazepine in adults. Epilepsia 1994;35:1026–8.
22. Parker AP, Agathonikou A, Robinson RO, Panayiotopoulos CP. Inappropriate use of carbamazepine and vigabatrin in typical absence seizures. Dev Med Child Neurol 1998;40:517–9.
23. Genton P, Gelisse P, Thomas P, Dravet C. Do carbamazepine and phenytoin aggravate juvenile myoclonic epilepsy? Neurology 2000;55:1106–9.
24. Thomas P, Valton L, Genton P. Absence and myoclonic status epilepticus precipitated by antiepileptic drugs in idiopathic generalized epilepsy. Brain 2006;129:1281–92.
25. Gayatri NA, Livingston JH. Aggravation of epilepsy by anti-epileptic drugs. Dev Med Child Neurol 2006;48:394–8.
26. Clobazam has equivalent efficacy to carbamazepine and phenytoin as monotherapy for childhood epilepsy. Canadian Study Group for Childhood Epilepsy. Epilepsia 1998;39:952–9.
27. Montenegro MA, Cendes F, Noronha AL, Mory SB, Carvalho MI, Marques LH, et al. Efficacy of clobazam as add-on therapy in patients with refractory partial epilepsy. Epilepsia 2001;42:539–42.
28. Sugai K. Clobazam as a new antiepileptic drug and clorazepate dipotassium as an alternative antiepileptic drug in Japan. Epilepsia 2004;45 Suppl:20–5.
29. Obeid T, Panayiotopoulos CP. Clonazepam in juvenile myoclonic epilepsy. Epilepsia 1989;30:603–6.
30. Oguni H, Uehara T, Tanaka T, Sunahara M, Hara M, Osawa M. Dramatic effect of ethosuximide on epileptic negative myoclonus: implications for the neurophysiological mechanism. Neuropediatrics 1998;29:29–34.
31. Guerrini R, Dravet C, Genton P, Belmonte A, Kaminska A, Dulac O. Lamotrigine and seizure aggravation in severe myoclonic epilepsy. Epilepsia 1998;39:508–12.
32. Guerrini R, Belmonte A, Parmeggiani L, Perucca E. Myoclonic status epilepticus following high-dosage lamotrigine therapy. Brain Dev 1999;21:420–4.
33. Biraben A, Allain H, Scarabin JM, Schuck S, Edan G. Exacerbation of juvenile myoclonic epilepsy with lamotrigine. Neurology 2000;55:1758.
34. Carrazana EJ, Wheeler SD. Exacerbation of juvenile myoclonic epilepsy with lamotrigine. Neurology 2001;56:1424–5.

35. Verrotti A, Domizio S, Franzoni E, Mohn A, Franzoni E, Coppola G et al. Levetiracetam in absence epilepsy: long-term efficacy in newly diagnosed patients. Dev Med Child Neurol 2008;50:850–3.
36. Di Bonaventura C, Fattouch J, Mari F, Egeo G, Vaudano AE, Prencipe M, et al. Clinical experience with levetiracetam in idiopathic generalized epilepsy according to different syndrome subtypes. Epileptic Disord 2005;7:231–5.
37. Kaddurah AK, Holmes GL. Possible precipitation of myoclonic seizures with oxcarbazepine. Epilepsy Behav 2006;8:289–93.
38. Gelisse P, Genton P, Kuate D, Pesenti A, Baldy-Moulinier M, Crespel A. Worsening of seizures by oxcarbazepine in juvenile idiopathic generalized epilepsies. Epilepsia 2004;45:1282–8.
39. Vendrame M, Khurana DS, Cruz M, Melvin J, Valencia I, Legido A, et al. Aggravation of seizures and/or EEG features in children treated with oxcarbazepine monotherapy. Epilepsia 2007;48:2116–20.
40. Huppertz HJ, Feuerstein TJ, Schulze-Bonhage A. Myoclonus in epilepsy patients with anticonvulsive add-on therapy with pregabalin. Epilepsia 2001;42:790–2.
41. Knake S, Klein KM, Hattemer K, Wellek A, Oertel WH, Hamer HM, et al. Pregabalin-induced generalized myoclonic status epilepticus in patients with chronic pain. Epilepsy Behav 2007;11:471–3.
42. Striano P, Coppola A, Madia F, Pezzella M, Ciampa C, Zara F, et al. Life-threatening status epilepticus following gabapentin administration in a patient with benign adult familial myoclonic epilepsy. Epilepsia 2007;48:1995–8.
43. Arzimanoglou A, Rahbani A. Zonisamide for the treatment of epilepsy. Expert Rev Neurother 2006;6:1283–92.
44. Glauser T, Ben-Menachem E, Bourgeois B, Cnaan A, Chadwick D, Guerreiro C, et al. ILAE treatment guidelines: evidence-based analysis of antiepileptic drug efficacy and effectiveness as initial monotherapy for epileptic seizures and syndromes. Epilepsia 2006;47:1094–120.
45. French JA. Now we know the drug of first choice – or do we? Epilepsy Curr 2007;7:125–7.
46. Gelisse P, Juntas-Morales R, Genton P, Hillaire-Buys D, Diaz O, Coubes P, et al. Dramatic weight loss with levetiracetam. Epilepsia 2008; 49:308–15.
47. Perucca E, Johannessen SI. The ideal pharmacokinetic properties of an antiepileptic drug: how close does levetiracetam come? Epileptic Disord 2003;5 Suppl 1:S17–26.
48. Patsalos PN. Properties of antiepileptic drugs in the treatment of idiopathic generalized epilepsies. Epilepsia 2005;46 Suppl 9:140–8.
49. Patsalos PN. Levetiracetam. Rev Contemp Pharm 2004;13:1–168.
50. Tran TA, Leppik IE, Blesi K, Sathanandan ST, Remmel R. Lamotrigine clearance during pregnancy. Neurology 2002;59:251–5.
51. Ferrie CD, Robinson RO, Knott C, Panayiotopoulos CP. Lamotrigine as an add-on drug in typical absence seizures. Acta Neurol Scand 1995;91:200–2.
52. Reutens DC, Duncan JS, Patsalos PN. Disabling tremor after lamotrigine with sodium valproate. Lancet 1993;342:185–6.
53. Morrow J, Russell A, Guthrie E, Parsons L, Robertson I, Waddell R, et al. Malformation risks of antiepileptic drugs in pregnancy: a prospective study from the UK Epilepsy and Pregnancy Register. J Neurol Neurosurg Psychiatry 2006;77:193–8.
54. Czapinski P, Blaszczyk B, Czuczwar SJ. Mechanisms of action of antiepileptic drugs. Curr Top Med Chem 2005;5:3–14.
55. Luszczki JJ. Third-generation antiepileptic drugs: mechanisms of action, pharmacokinetics and interactions. Pharmacol Rep 2009;61:197–216.
56. Stefan H, Feuerstein TJ. Novel anticonvulsant drugs. Pharmacol Ther 2007;113:165–83.
57. Bialer M, Johannessen SI, Levy RH, Perucca E, Tomson T, White HS. Progress report on new antiepileptic drugs: a summary of the Ninth Eilat Conference (EILAT IX). Epilepsy Res 2009;83:1–43.
58. Kaminski RM, Matagne A, Patsalos PN, Klitgaard H. Benefit of combination therapy in epilepsy: a review of the preclinical evidence with levetiracetam. Epilepsia 2009;50:387–97.
59. Deckers CL, Czuczwar SJ, Hekster YA, Keyser A, Kubova H, Meinardi H et al. Selection of antiepileptic drug polytherapy based on mechanisms of action: the evidence reviewed. Epilepsia 2000;41:1364–74.
60. Kwan P, Brodie MJ. Combination therapy in epilepsy: when and what to use. Drugs 2006;66:1817–29.
61. Cross SA, Curran MP. Lacosamide: in partial-onset seizures. Drugs 2009;69:449–59.
62. Privitera MD, Brodie MJ, Mattson RH, Chadwick DW, Neto W, Wang S. Topiramate, carbamazepine and valproate monotherapy: double-blind comparison in newly diagnosed epilepsy. Acta Neurol Scand 2003;107:165–75.
63. Kwan P, Brodie MJ. Effectiveness of first antiepileptic drug. Epilepsia 2001;42:1255–60.
64. Schiller Y, Najjar Y. Quantifying the response to antiepileptic drugs: effect of past treatment history. Neurology 2008;70:54–65.
65. Schmidt D, Elger C, Holmes GL. Pharmacological overtreatment in epilepsy: mechanisms and management. Epilepsy Res 2002;52:3–14.
66. Deckers CL, Knoester PD, de Haan GJ, Keyser A, Renier WO, Hekster YA. Selection criteria for the clinical use of the newer antiepileptic drugs. CNS Drugs 2003;17:405–21.

67. Lynch BA, Lambeng N, Nocka K, Kensel-Hammes P, Bajjalieh SM, Matagne A, et al. The synaptic vesicle protein SV2A is the binding site for the antiepileptic drug levetiracetam. Proc Natl Acad Sci USA 2004;101:9861–6.

68. Liow K. Understanding patients' perspective in the use of generic antiepileptic drugs: compelling lessons for physicians to improve physician/patient communication. BMC Neurol 2009;9:11.

69. Van PW, Hauman H, Lagae L. The use of generic medication in epilepsy: a review of potential issues and challenges. Eur J Paediatr Neurol 2009;13:87–92.

70. Berg MJ, Gross RA, Haskins LS, Zingaro WM, Tomaszewski KJ. Generic substitution in the treatment of epilepsy: patient and physician perceptions. Epilepsy Behav 2008;13:693–9.

71. Gidal BE, Tomson T. Debate: Substitution of generic drugs in epilepsy: is there cause for concern? Epilepsia 2008;49 Suppl 9:56–62.

72. Privitera MD. Generic antiepileptic drugs: current controversies and future directions. Epilepsy Curr 2008;8:113–7.

73. Andermann F, Duh MS, Gosselin A, Paradis PE. Compulsory generic switching of antiepileptic drugs: high switchback rates to branded compounds compared with other drug classes. Epilepsia 2007;48:464–9.

74. Heaney DC, Sander JW. Antiepileptic drugs: generic versus branded treatments. Lancet Neurol 2007;6:465–8.

75. Miller JW, Anderson GD, Doherty MJ, Poolos NP. Position statement on the coverage of anticonvulsant drugs for the treatment of epilepsy: what's the problem with generic antiepileptic drugs? A call to action. Neurology 2007;69:1806–8.

76. Bialer M. Generic products of antiepileptic drugs (AEDs): is it an issue? Epilepsia 2007;48:1825–32.

77. Bochner F, Hooper WD, Tyrer JH, Eadie MJ. Factors involved in an outbreak of phenytoin intoxication. J Neurol Sci 1972;16:481–7.

78. Patsalos PN, Berry DJ, Bourgeois BF, Cloyd JC, Glauser TA, Johannessen SI et al. Antiepileptic drugs--best practice guidelines for therapeutic drug monitoring: a position paper by the subcommission on therapeutic drug monitoring, ILAE Commission on Therapeutic Strategies. Epilepsia 2008;49:1239–76.

79. Shorvon S. We live in the age of the clinical guideline. Epilepsia 2006;47:1091–3.

80. Sackett DL, Rosenberg WM, Gray JA, Haynes RB, Richardson WS. Evidence based medicine: what it is and what it isn't. BMJ 1996;312:71–2.

81. Dickersin K, Straus SE, Bero LA. Evidence based medicine: increasing, not dictating, choice. BMJ 2007;334 Suppl 1:s10.

82. French JA. First-choice drug for newly diagnosed epilepsy. Lancet 2007;369:970–1.

83. French JA. Response: efficacy and tolerability of the new antiepileptic drugs. Epilepsia 2004;45:1649–51.

84. Marson AG, Al-Kharusi AM, Alwaidh M, Appleton R, Baker GA, Chadwick DW, et al. The SANAD study of effectiveness of valproate, lamotrigine, or topiramate for generalised and unclassifiable epilepsy: an unblinded randomised controlled trial. Lancet 2007;369:1016–26.

85. Marson AG, Williamson PR, Clough H, Hutton JL, Chadwick DW. Carbamazepine versus valproate monotherapy for epilepsy: a metaanalysis. Epilepsia 2002;43:505–13.

86. Chadwick D. Safety and efficacy of vigabatrin and carbamazepine in newly diagnosed epilepsy: a multicentre randomised doubleblind study. Vigabatrin European Monotherapy Study Group. Lancet 1999;354:13–9.

87. Eke T, Talbot JF, Lawden MC. Severe persistent visual field constriction associated with vigabatrin. BMJ 1997;314:180–1.

88. Panayiotopoulos CP, Benbadis SR, Covanis A, Dulac O, Duncan JS, Eeg-Olofsson O, et al. Efficacy and tolerability of the new antiepileptic drugs; commentary on the recently published practice parameters. Epilepsia 2004;45:1646–9.

89. Walker MC, Sander JW. Difficulties in extrapolating from clinical trial data to clinical practice: the case of antiepileptic drugs. Neurology 1997;49:333–7.

90. Beghi E. Efficacy and tolerability of the new antiepileptic drugs: comparison of two recent guidelines. Lancet Neurol 2004;3:618–21.

91. French JA, Kanner AM, Bautista J, Abou-Khalil B, Browne T, Harden CL, et al. Efficacy and tolerability of the new antiepileptic drugs I: treatment of new onset epilepsy: report of the Therapeutics and Technology Assessment Subcommittee and Quality Standards Subcommittee of the American Academy of Neurology and the American Epilepsy Society. Neurology 2004;62:1252–60.

92. Patsalos PN. Clinical pharmacokinetics of levetiracetam. Clin Pharmacokinet 2004;43:707–24.

93. Patsalos PN. The pharmacokinetic characteristics of levetiracetam. Methods Find Exp Clin Pharmacol 2003;25:123–9.

94. Brodie MJ, Perucca E, Ryvlin P, Ben-Menachem E, Meencke HJ. Comparison of levetiracetam and controlled-release carbamazepine in newly diagnosed epilepsy. Neurology 2007;68:402–8.

95. Berkovic SF, Knowlton RC, Leroy RF, Schiemann J, Falter U. Placebo-controlled study of levetiracetam in idiopathic generalized epilepsy. Neurology 2007;69:1751–60.

96. Guidelines for therapeutic monitoring on antiepileptic drugs. Commission on Antiepileptic Drugs, International League Against Epilepsy. Epilepsia 1993;34:585–7.

97. Johannessen SI, Tomson T. Pharmacokinetic variability of newer antiepileptic drugs: when is monitoring needed? Clin Pharmacokinet 2006;45:1061–75.

98. Glauser TA, Pippenger CE. Controversies in blood-level monitoring: reexamining its role in the treatment of epilepsy. Epilepsia 2000;41 Suppl 8:S6–15.
99. Battino D, Croci D, Rossini A, Messina S, Mamoli D, Perucca E.Topiramate pharmacokinetics in children and adults with epilepsy: a case-matched comparison based on therapeutic drug monitoring data. Clin Pharmacokinet 2005;44:407–16.
100. Johannessen SI, Battino D, Berry DJ, Bialer M, Kramer G, Tomson T et al. Therapeutic drug monitoring of the newer antiepileptic drugs.Ther Drug Monit 2003;25:347–63.
101. Jannuzzi G, Cian P, Fattore C, Gatti G, Bartoli A, Monaco F, et al. A multicenter randomized controlled trial on the clinical impact of therapeutic drug monitoring in patients with newly diagnosed epilepsy. The Italian TDM Study Group in Epilepsy. Epilepsia 2000;41:222–30.
102. Elzagallaai AA, Knowles SR, Rieder MJ, Bend JR, Shear NH, Koren G. In vitro testing for the diagnosis of anticonvulsant hypersensitivity syndrome: a systematic review. Mol Diagn Ther 2009;13:313–30.
103. Bohan KH, Mansuri TF, Wilson NM. Anticonvulsant hypersensitivity syndrome: implications for pharmaceutical care. Pharmacotherapy 2007;27:1425–39.
104. Cumbo-Nacheli G, Weinberger J, Alkhalil M, Thati N, Baptist AP. Anticonvulsant hypersensitivity syndrome: is there a role for immunomodulation? Epilepsia 2008;49:2108–12.
105. Elzagallaai AA, Knowles SR, Rieder MJ, Bend JR, Shear NH, Koren G. Patch testing for the diagnosis of anticonvulsant hypersensitivity syndrome: a systematic review. Drug Saf 2009;32:391–408.
106. Mansur AT, Pekcan YS, Goktay F. Anticonvulsant hypersensitivity syndrome: clinical and laboratory features. Int J Dermatol 2008;47:1184–9.
107. Sabroe TP, Sabers A. Progressive anticonvulsant hypersensitivity syndrome associated with change of drug product. Acta Neurol Scand 2008;117:428–31.
108. Seitz CS, Pfeuffer P, Raith P, Brocker EB, Trautmann A. Anticonvulsant hypersensitivity syndrome: cross-reactivity with tricyclic antidepressant agents. Ann Allergy Asthma Immunol 2006;97:698–702.
109. Ting TY. Anticonvulsant hypersensitivity syndrome: identification and management. Curr Treat Options Neurol 2007;9:243–8.
110. US Food and Drug Administration. Dangerous or even fatal skin reactions: carbamazepine (marketed as Carbatrol, Equetro, Tegretol, and generics). Available online at http://www.fda.gov/Drugs/ DrugSafety/ PostmarketDrugSafetyInformationforPatientsandProviders/ ucm124718.htm. Last accessed 27 November 2009.
111. US Food and Drug Administration. Suicidal behavior and ideation and antiepileptic drugs. Available online at http://www.fda.gov/Drugs/ DrugSafety/PostmarketDrugSafetyInformationforPatientsandProviders/ ucm100192.htm Last accessed 27 November 2009.
112. Bell GS, Sander JW. Suicide and epilepsy. Curr Opin Neurol 2009;22:174–8.
113. Bell GS, Mula M, Sander JW. Suicidality in people taking antiepileptic drugs: What is the evidence? CNS Drugs 2009;23:281–92.
114. Kanner AM. Depression in epilepsy: a complex relation with unexpected consequences. Curr Opin Neurol 2008;21:190–4.
115. Mula M, Sander JW. Suicidal ideation in epilepsy and levetiracetam therapy. Epilepsy Behav 2007;11:130–2.
116. Kanner AM. Depression and epilepsy: A new perspective on two closely related disorders. Epilepsy Curr 2006;6:141–6.
117. Zaccara G, Balestieri F, Ragazzoni A. Management of side effects of antiepileptic dugs. In: Shorvon S, Perucca E, Engel JJr, eds. The treatment of epilepsy (3nd edition). Philadelphia: Wiley-Blackwell, 2009:289–99.
118. Zaccara G, Gangemi PF, Cincotta M. Central nervous system adverse effects of new antiepileptic drugs. A meta-analysis of placebo-controlled studies. Seizure 2008;17:405–21.
119. Arif H, Buchsbaum R, Weintraub D, Pierro J, Resor SR, Jr., Hirsch LJ. Patient-reported cognitive side effects of antiepileptic drugs: predictors and comparison of all commonly used antiepileptic drugs. Epilepsy Behav 2009;14:202–9.
120. Mula M, Trimble MR. Antiepileptic drug-induced cognitive adverse effects: potential mechanisms and contributing factors. CNS Drugs 2009;23:121–37.
121. Taylor J, Kolamunnage-Dona R, Marson AG, Smith PE, Aldenkamp AP, Baker GA. Patients with epilepsy: cognitively compromised before the start of antiepileptic drug treatment? Epilepsia 2010;51:48–56.
122. Berg AT, Langfitt JT, Testa FM, Levy SR, DiMario F, Westerveld M et al. Global cognitive function in children with epilepsy: a community-based study. Epilepsia 2008;49:608–14.
123. Helmstaedter C, Witt JA. The effects of levetiracetam on cognition: a non-interventional surveillance study. Epilepsy Behav 2008;13:642–9.
124. Kanner AM. Can antiepileptic drugs unmask a susceptibility to psychiatric disorders? Nat Clin Pract Neurol 2009;5:132–3.
125. Mula M, Trimble MR, Sander JW. Are psychiatric adverse events of antiepileptic drugs a unique entity? A study on topiramate and levetiracetam. Epilepsia 2007;48:2322–6.
126. Weintraub D, Buchsbaum R, Resor SR, Jr., Hirsch LJ. Psychiatric and behavioral side effects of the newer antiepileptic drugs in adults with epilepsy. Epilepsy Behav 2007;10:105–10.
127. Gilliam FG, Santos JM. Adverse psychiatric effects of antiepileptic drugs. Epilepsy Res 2006;68:67–9.

128. Besag FM. Behavioural effects of the newer antiepileptic drugs: an update. Expert Opin Drug Saf 2004;3:1–8.

129. Glauser TA. Effects of antiepileptic medications on psychiatric and behavioral comorbidities in children and adolescents with epilepsy. Epilepsy Behav 2004;5 Suppl 3:S25–S32.

130. Trimble MR, Rusch N, Betts T, Crawford PM. Psychiatric symptoms after therapy with new antiepileptic drugs: psychopathological and seizure related variables. Seizure 2000;9:249–54.

131. Schmitz B. Psychiatric syndromes related to antiepileptic drugs. Epilepsia 1999;40 Suppl 10:S65–S70.

132. Elliott B, Amarouche M, Shorvon SD. Psychiatric features of epilepsy and their management. In: Shorvon S, Perucca E, Engel JJr, eds. The treatment of epilepsy, 3rd edition, pp 273–87. Philadelphia: Wiley-Blackwell.

133. Ettinger AB, Argoff CE. Use of antiepileptic drugs for nonepileptic conditions: psychiatric disorders and chronic pain. Neurotherapeutics 2007;4:75–83.

134. Clemens B. Forced normalisation precipitated by lamotrigine. Seizure 2005;14:485–9.

135. Witchel HJ, Hancox JC, Nutt DJ. Psychotropic drugs, cardiac arrhythmia, and sudden death. J Clin Psychopharmacol 2003;23:58–77.

136. Woosley RL. Drugs that prolong the QT interval and/or induce Torsades de Pointes. Available online at http://www.azcert.org/medicalpros/ drug-lists/printable-drug-list.cfm. Last accessed 27 November 2009.

137. Singh G. Management of medical co-morbidity associated with epilepsy. In: Shorvon S, Perucca E, Engel JJr, eds. The treatment of epilepsy, 3nd edition, pp 268–9. Philadelphia: Wiley-Blackwell, 2009.

138. Holbrook M, Malik M, Shah RR, Valentin JP. Drug induced shortening of the QT/QTc interval: an emerging safety issue warranting further modelling and evaluation in drug research and development? J Pharmacol Toxicol Methods 2009;59:21–8.

139. DeSilvey DL, Moss AJ. Primidone in the treatment of the long QT syndrome: QT shortening and ventricular arrhythmia suppression. Ann Intern Med 1980;93:53–4.

140. Christidis D, Kalogerakis D, Chan TY, Mauri D, Alexiou G, Terzoudi A. Is primidone the drug of choice for epileptic patients with QT-prolongation? A comprehensive analysis of literature. Seizure 2006;15:64–6.

141. Shah RR. Cardiac effects of antiepileptic drugs. In: Panayiotopoulos CP, ed. Atlas of epilepsies (in press). London: Springer, 2010.

142. Erikssen J, Otterstad JE. Natural course of a prolonged PR interval and the relation between PR and incidence of coronary heart disease. A 7-year follow-up study of 1832 apparently healthy men aged 40-59 years. Clin Cardiol 1984;7:6–13.

143. Matsuo F, Bergen D, Faught E, Messenheimer JA, Dren AT, Rudd GD et al. Placebo-controlled study of the efficacy and safety of lamotrigine in patients with partial seizures. U.S. Lamotrigine Protocol 0.5 Clinical Trial Group. Neurology 1993;43:2284–91.

144. French JA, Kanner AM, Bautista J, Abou-Khalil B, Browne T, Harden CL et al. Efficacy and tolerability of the new antiepileptic drugs I: treatment of new onset epilepsy: report of the Therapeutics and Technology Assessment Subcommittee and Quality Standards Subcommittee of the American Academy of Neurology and the American Epilepsy Society. Neurology 2004;62:1252–60.

145. French JA, Kanner AM, Bautista J, Abou-Khalil B, Browne T, Harden CL et al. Efficacy and tolerability of the new antiepileptic drugs II: treatment of refractory epilepsy: report of the Therapeutics and Technology Assessment Subcommittee and Quality Standards Subcommittee of the American Academy of Neurology and the American Epilepsy Society. Neurology 2004;62:1261–73.

146. Tomson T, Kenneback G. Arrhythmia, heart rate variability, and antiepileptic drugs. Epilepsia 1997;38:S48-S51.

147. Saetre E, Abdelnoor M, Amlie JP, Tossebro M, Perucca E, Taubøll E et al. Cardiac function and antiepileptic drug treatment in the elderly: A comparison between lamotrigine and sustained-release carbamazepine. Epilepsia 2009; 50:1841–9.

148. Saetre E, Perucca E, Isojarvi J, Gjerstad L. An international multicenter randomized double-blind controlled trial of lamotrigine and sustained-release carbamazepine in the treatment of newly diagnosed epilepsy in the elderly. Epilepsia 2007;48:1292–302.

149. Danielsson BR, Lansdell K, Patmore L, Tomson T. Effects of the antiepileptic drugs lamotrigine, topiramate and gabapentin on hERG potassium currents. Epilepsy Res 2005;63:17–25.

150. Brown AM. HERG block, QT liability and sudden cardiac death. Novartis Found Symp 2005;266:118–31.

151. Sanguinetti MC, Tristani-Firouzi M. hERG potassium channels and cardiac arrhythmia. Nature 2006;440:463–9.

152. Aurlien D, Taubøll E, Gjerstad L. Lamotrigine in idiopathic epilepsy - increased risk of cardiac death? Acta Neurol Scand 2007;115:199–203.

153. Aurlien D, Leren TP, Taubøll E, Gjerstad L. New SCN5A mutation in a SUDEP victim with idiopathic epilepsy. Seizure 2009;18:158–60.

154. Danielsson C, Azarbayjani F, Skold AC, Sjogren N, Danielsson BR. Polytherapy with hERG-blocking antiepileptic drugs: increased risk for embryonic cardiac arrhythmia and teratogenicity. Birth Defects Res A Clin Mol Teratol 2007;79:595–603.

155. Panayiotopoulos CP, Crawford P, Tomson T, (eds). Volume 4: Epilepsies in girls and women. Oxford: Medicinae, 2008.

156. Morrow J. The XX factor. Treating women with anti-epileptic drugs. Cressing, Essex: National Services for Helth Improvement, 2007.
157. Harden CL, Pennell PB, Koppel BS, Hovinga CA, Gidal B, Meador KJ et al. Practice parameter update: management issues for women with epilepsy--focus on pregnancy (an evidence-based review): vitamin K, folic acid, blood levels, and breastfeeding: report of the Quality Standards Subcommittee and Therapeutics and Technology Assessment Subcommittee of the American Academy of Neurology and American Epilepsy Society. Neurology 2009;73:142–9.
158. Harden CL, Meador KJ, Pennell PB, Hauser WA, Gronseth GS, French JA et al. Practice parameter update: management issues for women with epilepsy--focus on pregnancy (an evidence-based review): teratogenesis and perinatal outcomes: report of the Quality Standards Subcommittee and Therapeutics and Technology Assessment Subcommittee of the American Academy of Neurology and American Epilepsy Society. Neurology 2009;73:133–41.
159. Harden CL, Hopp J, Ting TY, Pennell PB, French JA, Hauser WA et al. Practice parameter update: management issues for women with epilepsy--focus on pregnancy (an evidence-based review): obstetrical complications and change in seizure frequency: report of the Quality Standards Subcommittee and Therapeutics and Technology Assessment Subcommittee of the American Academy of Neurology and American Epilepsy Society. Neurology 2009;73:126–32.
160. Aguglia U, Barboni G, Battino D, Cavazzuti GB, Citernesi A, Corosu R et al. Italian consensus conference on epilepsy and pregnancy, labor and puerperium. Epilepsia 2009;50 Suppl 1:7–23.
161. Vajda FJ. Treatment options for pregnant women with epilepsy. Expert Opin Pharmacother 2008;9:1859–68.
162. Battino D, Tomson T. Management of epilepsy during pregnancy. Drugs 2007;67:2727–46.
163. Tomson T, Battino D, French J, Harden C, Holmes L, Morrow J et al. Antiepileptic drug exposure and major congenital malformations: the role of pregnancy registries. Epilepsy Behav 2007;11:277–82.
164. Tomson T, Hiilesmaa V. Epilepsy in pregnancy. BMJ 2007;335:769-73.
165. Perucca E. Birth defects after prenatal exposure to antiepileptic drugs. Lancet Neurol 2005;4:781–6.
166. Tomson T, Battino D. Pregnancy and epilepsy: what should we tell our patients? J Neurol 2009;256:856–62.
167. Walker SP, Permezel M, Berkovic SF. The management of epilepsy in pregnancy. BJOG 2009;116:758–67.
168. Beach RL, Kaplan PW. Seizures in pregnancy: diagnosis and management. Int Rev Neurobiol 2008;83:259–71.
169. Brodtkorb E, Reimers A. Seizure control and pharmacokinetics of antiepileptic drugs in pregnant women with epilepsy. Seizure 2008;17:160–5.
170. Pennell PB, Hovinga CA. Antiepileptic drug therapy in pregnancy I: gestation-induced effects on AED pharmacokinetics. Int Rev Neurobiol 2008;83:227-40.
171. Pennell PB. Antiepileptic drugs during pregnancy: what is known and which AEDs seem to be safest? Epilepsia 2008;49 Suppl 9:43–55.
172. Pennell PB, Peng L, Newport DJ, Ritchie JC, Koganti A, Holley DK et al. Lamotrigine in pregnancy: clearance, therapeutic drug monitoring, and seizure frequency. Neurology 2008;70:2130–6.
173. Robinson JN, Cleary-Goldman J. Management of epilepsy and pregnancy: an obstetrical perspective. Int Rev Neurobiol 2008;83:273–82.
174. Tomson T, Crawford P. Practical pre-pregnancy counselling. In: Panayiotopoulos CP, Crawford P, Tomson T, eds. Volume 4: Epilepsies in girls and women. Oxford: Medicinae, 2008:170–3.
175. Kaplan PW, Norwitz ER, Ben-Menachem E, Pennell PB, Druzin M, Robinson JN et al. Obstetric risks for women with epilepsy during pregnancy. Epilepsy Behav 2007;11:283–91.
176. Crawford PM. Managing epilepsy in women of childbearing age. Drug Saf 2009;32:293–307.
177. Meador KJ, Pennell PB, Harden CL, Gordon JC, Tomson T, Kaplan PW et al. Pregnancy registries in epilepsy: a consensus statement on health outcomes. Neurology 2008;71:1109–17.
178. Battino D, Tomson T. The management of epilepsy in pregnancy. In: Shorvon S, Pedley TA, eds. The epilepsies 3, pp :241–64. Philadelphia: Saunders, Elsevier, 2008.
179. Sabers A. Interactions between anti-epileptic drugs and hormonal contraception. In: Panayiotopoulos CP, Crawford P, Tomson T, eds. Volume 4: Epilepsies in girls and women, pp 93–7. Oxford: Medicinae, 2008.
180. Dutton C, Foldvary-Schaefer N. Contraception in women with epilepsy: pharmacokinetic interactions, contraceptive options, and management. Int Rev Neurobiol 2008;83:113–34.
181. O'Brien MD, Guillebaud J. Contraception for women with epilepsy. Epilepsia 2006;47:1419–22.
182. Adab N, Kini U, Vinten J, Ayres J, Baker G, Clayton-Smith J. The longer term outcome of children born to mothers with epilepsy. J Neurol Neurosurg Psychiatry 2004;75:1575–83.
183. Johannessen LC, Patsalos PN. Pharmacokinetics of AEDs in pregnancy. In: Panayiotopoulos CP, Crawford P, Tomson T, eds. Volume 4: Epilepsies in girls and women. Oxford: Medicinae, 2008:143–9.
184. Tomson T, Battino D. Pharmacokinetics and therapeutic drug monitoring of newer antiepileptic drugs during pregnancy and the puerperium. Clin Pharmacokinet 2007;46:209–19.
185. Lamictal® (lamotrigine). Product information (Australia). GlaxoSmithKline, 2009.
186. Palmieri C, Canger R. Teratogenic potential of the newer antiepileptic drugs: what is known and how should this influence prescribing? CNS Drugs 2002;16:755–64.

187. Holmes LB, Baldwin EJ, Smith CR, Habecker E, Glassman L, Wong SL et al. Increased frequency of isolated cleft palate in infants exposed to lamotrigine during pregnancy. Neurology 2008;70:2152–8.

188. Nelson K, Holmes LB. Malformations due to presumed spontaneous mutations in newborn infants. N Engl J Med 1989;320:19–23.

189. Cunnington M, Tennis P. Lamotrigine and the risk of malformations in pregnancy. Neurology 2005;64:955–60.

190. Honein MA, Paulozzi LJ, Cragan JD, Correa A. Evaluation of selected characteristics of pregnancy drug registries. Teratology 1999;60:356–64.

191. Hauser WA, Tomson T. Lamotrigine and the risk of malformations in pregnancy. Neurology 2006;66:153–4.

192. Morrow J, Russell A, Guthrie E, Parsons L, Robertson I, Waddell R et al. Malformation risks of antiepileptic drugs in pregnancy: a prospective study from the UK Epilepsy and Pregnancy Register. J Neurol Neurosurg Psychiatry 2006;77:193–8.

193. Meador KJ, Baker GA, Browning N, Clayton-Smith J, Combs-Cantrell DT, Cohen M et al. Cognitive function at 3 years of age after fetal exposure to antiepileptic drugs. N Engl J Med 2009;360:1597–605.

194. Practice parameter: management issues for women with epilepsy (summary statement). Report of the Quality Standards Subcommittee of the American Academy of Neurology. Neurology 1998;51:944–8.

195. McElhatton PR. The effects of benzodiazepine use during pregnancy and lactation. Reprod Toxicol 1994;8:461–75.

196. Diaz-Romero RM, Garza-Morales S, Mayen-Molina DG, Ibarra-Puig J, Avila-Rosas H. Facial anthropometric measurements in offspring of epileptic mothers. Arch Med Res 1999;30:186–9.

197. Eros E, Czeizel AE, Rockenbauer M, Sorensen HT, Olsen J. A population-based case-control teratologic study of nitrazepam, medazepam, tofisopam, alprazolum and clonazepam treatment during pregnancy. Eur J Obstet Gynecol Reprod Biol 2002;101:147–54.

198. Lin AE, Peller AJ, Westgate MN, Houde K, Franz A, Holmes LB. Clonazepam use in pregnancy and the risk of malformations. Birth Defects Res A Clin Mol Teratol 2004;70:534–6.

199. Hunt SJ, Craig JJ, Morrow JI. Increased frequency of isolated cleft palate in infants exposed to lamotrigine during pregnancy. Neurology 2009;72:1108–9.

200. Dolk H, Jentink J, Loane M, Morris J, de Jong-van den Berg LT. Does lamotrigine use in pregnancy increase orofacial cleft risk relative to other malformations? Neurology 2008;71:714–22.

201. Eurap Study Group. Utilization of antiepileptic drugs during pregnancy: comparative patterns in 38 countries based on data from the EURAP registry. Epilepsia 2009;50:2305–9.

202. Hunt S, Craig J, Russell A, Guthrie E, Parsons L, Robertson I et al. Levetiracetam in pregnancy: preliminary experience from the UK Epilepsy and Pregnancy Register. Neurology 2006;67:1876–9.

203. Ornoy A, Zvi N, Arnon J, Wajnberg R, Shechtman S, Diav-Citrin O. The outcome of pregnancy following topiramate treatment: a study on 52 pregnancies. Reprod Toxicol 2008;25:388–9.

204. Hunt S, Russell A, Smithson WH, Parsons L, Robertson I, Waddell R et al. Topiramate in pregnancy: preliminary experience from the UK Epilepsy and Pregnancy Register. Neurology 2008;71:272–6.

205. Fountain NB. A pregnant pause to consider teratogenicity of topiramate. Epilepsy Curr 2009;9:36–8.

206. Petrenaite V, Sabers A, Hansen-Schwartz J. Seizure deterioration in women treated with oxcarbazepine during pregnancy. Epilepsy Res 2009;84:245–9.

207. Ng YT. The fetal anticonvulsant syndrome. In: Gilman S, ed. Medlink Neurology. San Diego SA: Arbor Publishing Corp, 2009.

208. The EURAP study group. Seizure control and treatment in pregnancy: observations from the EURAP epilepsy pregnancy registry. Neurology 2006;66:354–60.

209. Battino D, Tomson T. Seizure control in pregnancy. In: Panayiotopoulos CP, Crawford P, Tomson T, eds. Volume 4: Epilepsies in girls and women. Oxford: Medicinae, 2008:138–42.

210. Janz D. Die epilepsien:Spezielle pathologie und therapie. Stuttgart: Georg Thieme, 1969.

211. Shorvon SD. Status epilepticus: its clinical features and treatment in children and adults. Cambridge: Cambridge University Press, 1994.

212. Vajda FJ, Hitchcock A, Graham J, Solinas C, O'Brien TJ, Lander CM et al. Foetal malformations and seizure control: 52 months data of the Australian Pregnancy Registry. Eur J Neurol 2006;13:645–54.

213. Johannessen SI, Tomson T. Pharmacokinetic variability of newer antiepileptic drugs: when is monitoring needed? Clin Pharmacokinet 2006;45:1061–75.

214. Pennell PB, Peng L, Newport DJ, Ritchie JC, Koganti A, Holley DK et al. Lamotrigine in pregnancy: clearance, therapeutic drug monitoring, and seizure frequency. Neurology 2008;70:2130–6.

215. Adab N, Tudur SC, Vinten J, Williamson P, Winterbottom J. Common antiepileptic drugs in pregnancy in women with epilepsy. Cochrane Database Syst Rev 2004;CD004848.

216. Zahn CA, Morrell MJ, Collins SD, Labiner DM, Yerby MS. Management issues for women with epilepsy: a review of the literature. Neurology 1998;51:949–56.

217. Morrow JI, Hunt SJ, Russell AJ, Smithson WH, Parsons L, Robertson I et al. Folic acid use and major congenital malformations in offspring of women with epilepsy: a prospective study from the UK Epilepsy and Pregnancy Register. J Neurol Neurosurg Psychiatry 2009;80:506–11.

218. Johannessen SI, Tomson T. Anti-epileptic drugs and breastfeeding. In: Panayiotopoulos CP, Crawford P, Tomson T, eds. Volume 4: Epilepsies in girls and women. Oxford: Medicinae, 2008:156–63.

219. Sabers A, Tomson T. Managing antiepileptic drugs during pregnancy and lactation. Curr Opin Neurol 2009;22:157–61.

220. Spencer JP, Gonzalez LS, III, Barnhart DJ. Medications in the breastfeeding mother. Am Fam Physician 2001;64:119–26.

221. Kooper AJ, de BD, van Ravenwaaij-Arts CM, Faas BH, Creemers JW, Thomas CM et al. Fetal anomaly scan potentially will replace routine AFAFP assays for the detection of neural tube defects. Prenat Diagn 2007;27:29–33.

222. Leppik IE. Treatment of epilepsy in the elderly. Curr Treat Options Neurol 2008;10:239–45.

223. Sirven JI. Treatment of the elderly with epilepsy. In: French JA, Delanty N, eds. Therapeutic Strategies in Epilepsy. Oxford: Clinical Publishing, 2009:173–85.

224. Mendiratta A, Pedley TA. Seizures and epilepsy in the edlerly. In: Shorvon S, Pedley TA, eds. The epilepsies 3. Philadelphia: Saunders, Elsevier, 2009:177–93.

225. Cloyd J, Hauser W, Towne A, Ramsay R, Mattson R, Gilliam F et al. Epidemiological and medical aspects of epilepsy in the elderly. Epilepsy Res 2006;68 Suppl 1:S39–S48.

226. Ramsay RE, Macias FM, Rowan AJ. Diagnosing epilepsy in the elderly. Int Rev Neurobiol 2007;81:129–51.

227. Leppik IE. Introduction to the International Geriatric Epilepsy Symposium (IGES). Epilepsy Res 2006;68 Suppl 1:S1–S4.

228. Brodie MJ, Stephen LJ. Outcomes in elderly patients with newly diagnosed and treated epilepsy. Int Rev Neurobiol 2007;81:253–63.

229. Sheth RD, Drazkowski JF, Sirven JI, Gidal BE, Hermann BP. Protracted ictal confusion in elderly patients. Arch Neurol 2006;63:529–32.

230. Thomas P, Beaumanoir A, Genton P, Dolisi C, Chatel M. 'De novo' absence status of late onset: report of 11 cases [see comments]. Neurology 1992;42:104–10.

231. Perucca E, Berlowitz D, Birnbaum A, Cloyd JC, Garrard J, Hanlon JT et al. Pharmacological and clinical aspects of antiepileptic drug use in the elderly. Epilepsy Res 2006;68 Suppl 1:S49–S63.

232. Bergey GK. Initial treatment of epilepsy: special issues in treating the elderly. Neurology 2004;63:S40–S48.

233. Patsalos PN. Anti-Epileptic Drug Interactions: A Clinical Guide. Cranleigh, U.K.: Clarius Press Ltd; 2005.

234. Leppik IE, Brodie MJ, Saetre ER, Rowan AJ, Ramsay RE, Jacobs MP. Outcomes research: clinical trials in the elderly. Epilepsy Res 2006;68 Suppl 1:S71–S76.

235. Leppik I. Antiepileptic drug trials in the elderly. Epilepsy Res 2006;68:45–8.

236. Rowan AJ, Ramsay RE, Collins JF, Pryor F, Boardman KD, Uthman BM et al. New onset geriatric epilepsy: a randomized study of gabapentin, lamotrigine, and carbamazepine. Neurology 2005;64:1868–73.

237. Brodie MJ, Overstall PW, Giorgi L. Multicentre, double-blind, randomised comparison between lamotrigine and carbamazepine in elderly patients with newly diagnosed epilepsy. The UK Lamotrigine Elderly Study Group. Epilepsy Res 1999;37:81–7.

238. Engel J, Jr., Wiebe S, French J, Sperling M, Williamson P, Spencer D, et al. Practice parameter: temporal lobe and localized neocortical resections for epilepsy: report of the Quality Standards Subcommittee of the American Academy of Neurology, in association with the American Epilepsy Society and the American Association of Neurological Surgeons. Neurology 2003;60:538–47.

239. Polkey CE. Clinical outcome of epilepsy surgery. Curr Opin Neurol 2004;17:173–8.

240. Tellez-Zenteno JF, Dhar R, Wiebe S. Long-term seizure outcomes following epilepsy surgery: a systematic review and meta-analysis. Brain 2005;128 Pt 5:1188–98.

241. Hirsch E, Arzimanoglou A. [Children with drug-resistant partial epilepsy: criteria for the identification of surgical candidates.] Rev Neurol (Paris) 2004;160:5S210–9.

242. Cross JH, Jayakar P, Nordli D, Delalande O, Duchowny M, Wieser HG, et al. Proposed criteria for referral and evaluation of children for epilepsy surgery: recommendations of the Subcommission for Pediatric Epilepsy Surgery. Epilepsia 2006;47:952–9.

243. Berg AT. Understanding the delay before epilepsy surgery: who develops intractable focal epilepsy and when? CNS Spectr 2004;9:136–44.

244. Shorvon S, Perucca E, Engel J.Jr. The treatment of epilepsy (third edition). In: Shorvon S, Perucca E, Engel J.Jr, eds. The treatment of epilepsy, 3rd edition, pp. 1–1056. Philadelphia: Wiley-Blackwell, 2009.

245. Wieser HG, Blume WT, Fish D, Goldensohn E, Hufnagel A, King D, et al. ILAE Commission Report. Proposal for a new classification of outcome with respect to epileptic seizures following epilepsy surgery. Epilepsia 2001;42:282–6.

246. Berg AT, Kelly MM. Defining intractability: comparisons among published definitions. Epilepsia 2006;47:431–6.

247. Berg AT, Vickrey BG, Testa FM, Levy SR, Shinnar S, DiMario F, et al. How long does it take for epilepsy to become intractable? A prospective investigation. Ann Neurol 2006;60:73–9.

248. Engel J, Jr. Surgery for seizures. N Engl J Med 1996;334:647–52.

249. Wheatley BM. Palliative surgery for intractable epilepsy. Adv Neurol 2006;97:549–56.

250. Morrell F, Whisler WW, Smith MC, Hoeppner TJ, de Toledo-Morrell L, Pierre-Louis SJ, et al. Landau-Kleffner syndrome. Treatment with subpial intracortical transection. Brain 1995;118 Pt 6:1529–46.

251. Morrell F, Kanner AM, Toledo-Morrell L, Hoeppner T, Whisler WW. Multiple subpial transection. Adv Neurol 1999;81:259–70. of Neurology and the American Epilepsy Society. Neurology 2004;62:1252–60.

252. Heck C, Helmers SL, DeGiorgio CM. Vagus nerve stimulation therapy, epilepsy, and device parameters: scientific basis and recommendations for use. Neurology 2002;59 Suppl 4:S31–7.

253. Privitera MD, Welty TE, Ficker DM, Welge J. Vagus nerve stimulation for partial seizures. Cochrane Database Syst Rev 2002;(1):CD002896.

254. Schachter SC. Vagus nerve stimulation: where are we? Curr Opin Neurol 2002;15:201–6.

255. Labar D. Vagus nerve stimulation for 1 year in 269 patients on unchanged antiepileptic drugs. Seizure 2004;13:392–8.

256. Tecoma ES, Iragui VJ. Vagus nerve stimulation use and effect in epilepsy: what have we learned? Epilepsy Behav 2006;8:127–36.

257. Boon P, Vonck K, De Reuck J, Caemaert J. Vagus nerve stimulation for refractory epilepsy. Seizure 2002;11 Suppl A:448–55.

258. Ben Menachem E. Vagus-nerve stimulation for the treatment of epilepsy. Lancet Neurol 2002;1:477–82.

259. Parker AP, Polkey CE, Binnie CD, Madigan C, Ferrie CD, Robinson RO. Vagal nerve stimulation in epileptic encephalopathies. Pediatrics 1999;103 Pt 1:778–82.

260. Parker AP, Polkey CE, Robinson RO. Vagal nerve stimulation in the epileptic encephalopathies: 3-year follow-up. Pediatrics 2001;108:221.

261. Kossoff EH, Pyzik PL, Rubenstein JE, Bergqvist AG, Buchhalter JR, Donner EJ, et al. Combined ketogenic diet and vagus nerve stimulation: rational polytherapy? Epilepsia 2007;48:77–81.

262. Freeman JM, Kossoff EH, Hartman AL. The ketogenic diet: one decade later. Pediatrics 2007;119:535–43.

263. Nordli D. The ketogenic diet: uses and abuses. Neurology 2002;58 Suppl 7:S21–4.

264. Hartman AL, Vining EP. Clinical aspects of the ketogenic diet. Epilepsia 2007;48:31–42.

265. Levy R, Cooper P. Ketogenic diet for epilepsy. Cochrane Database Syst Rev 2003;(3):CD001903.

266. Mackay MT, Bicknell-Royle J, Nation J, Humphrey M, Harvey AS. The ketogenic diet in refractory childhood epilepsy. J Paediatr Child Health 2005;41:353–7.

267. Bough KJ, Rho JM. Anticonvulsant mechanisms of the ketogenic diet. Epilepsia 2007;48:43–58.

268. Sinha SR, Kossoff EH. The ketogenic diet. Neurologist 2005;11:161– 70.

269. Villeneuve N, Pinton F, Bahi-Buisson N, Dulac O, Chiron C, Nabbout R. The ketogenic diet improves recently worsened focal epilepsy. Dev Med Child Neurol 2009;51:276–81.

270. Baranano KW, Hartman AL. The ketogenic diet: uses in epilepsy and other neurologic illnesses. Curr Treat Options Neurol 2008;10:410-9.

271. Kim dY, Rho JM. The ketogenic diet and epilepsy. Curr Opin Clin Nutr Metab Care 2008;11:113–20.

272. Neal EG, Chaffe H, Schwartz RH, Lawson MS, Edwards N, Fitzsimmons G et al. The ketogenic diet for the treatment of childhood epilepsy: a randomised controlled trial. Lancet Neurol 2008;7:500–6.

273. Stafstrom CE, Zupec-Kania B, Rho JM (eds). Ketogenic diet and related dietary treatments. Epilepsia 2008; 49(Suppl 8):1–133.

274. Coman DJ, Sinclair KG, Burke CJ, Appleton DB, Pelekanos JT, O'Neil CM, et al. Seizures, ataxia, developmental delay and the general paediatrician: glucose transporter 1 deficiency syndrome. J Paediatr Child Health 2006;42:263–7.

275. Wirrell EC, Darwish HZ, Williams-Dyjur C, Blackman M, Lange V. Is a fast necessary when initiating the ketogenic diet? J Child Neurol 2002;17:179–82.

276. Kossoff EH. More fat and fewer seizures: dietary therapies for epilepsy. Lancet Neurol 2004;3:415–20.

277. Kang HC, Lee HS, You SJ, Kang du C, Ko TS, Kim HD. Use of a modified Atkins diet in intractable childhood epilepsy. Epilepsia 2007;48:182–6.

278. Kossoff EH, Turner Z, Bluml RM, Pyzik PL, Vining EP. A randomized, crossover comparison of daily carbohydrate limits using the modified Atkins diet. Epilepsy Behav 2007;10:432–6.

279. Gupta R, Appleton R. Corticosteroids in the management of the paediatric epilepsies. Arch Dis Child 2005;90:379–84.

280. Gayatri N, Ferrie C, Cross H. Corticosteroids including ACTH for childhood epilepsy other than epileptic spasms. Cochrane Database Syst Rev 2007;(1):CD005222.

281. Buzatu M, Bulteau C, Altuzarra C, Dulac O, Van BP. Corticosteroids as treatment of epileptic syndromes with continuous spike-waves during slow-wave sleep. Epilepsia 2009;50 Suppl 7:68–72.

282. Panayiotopoulos CP. Epileptic syndromes and their treatment. London: Springer, 2010.

Index

Page numbers followed by **b** indicate boxes, page numbers followed by **f** indicate figures, and page numbers followed by **t** indicate tables.